A. Cesarani D. Alpini

Vertigo and Dizziness Rehabilitation

Springer

Berlin
Heidelberg
New York
Barcelona
Hong Kong
London
Milan
Paris
Singapore
Tokyo

Antonio Cesarani   Dario Alpini

Vertigo and Dizziness Rehabilitation

The MCS Method

With a contribution by C.-F. Claussen

Drawings by F. Alpini

With 173 Illustrations and 5 Tables

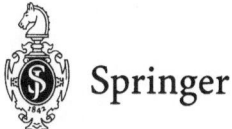 Springer

Antonio Cesarani, M.D.
Institute of Otolaryngology
University of Sassari
Via Mancini 5
17100 Sassari, Italy

Dario Alpini, M.D.
Centro Medico Sociale "S. Maria Nascente"
Don Carlo Gnocchi Foundation
ENT-Otoneurology Service
Via Capecelatro 66
20148 Milan, Italy

Dr. Claus-Frenz Claussen
President of the Neurotology and Equilibriometric Society
Kurhausstrasse 12
97688 Bad Kissingen, Germany

ISBN-13: 978-3-540-64084-4   e-ISBN-13: 978-3-642-59875-3
DOI: 10.1007/978-3-642-59875-3

Library of Congress Cataloging-in-Publication Data
Cesarani, A. (Antonio)
   Vertigo and dizziness rehabilitation: the MCS method / Antonio Cesarani, Dario Alpini; with a contri-
bution by C.-F. Claussen; drawings by F. Alpini.
   Includes bibliographical references and index.
ISBN-13: 978-3-540-64084-4
   1. Vertigo–Patients–Rehabilitation. 2. Dizziness–Patients–Rehabilitation. 3. Equilibrium (Physiology).
4. Vestibular apparatus–Diseases. I. Alpini, Dario, 1958– . II. Claussen, Claus-Frenz. III. Title.
   RF260.C47 1999
   616.8'41–ddc21

Illustrators: Regine Gattung-Petith and Albert P. Gattung, Edingen-Neckarhausen
Cover design: Künkel + Lopka Werbeagentur GmbH, Heidelberg
Typesetting: K+V Fotosatz GmbH, Beerfelden

SPIN: 10664717   21/3133-5 4 3 2 1 0 –

Preface

This volume opens a new frontier for clinical specialists dealing with vertigo sufferers. As our populations are constantly growing older, we have to deal more and more with degenerative neurosensorial disorders of elderly persons not only from the investigative, but also from the innovative therapeutic point of view.

This book's theme of vertigo and dizziness rehabilitation has been chosen in the sense of applied neurootometry and conservative neuroototherapy. The authors describe a new way of utilizing objective and quantitative neurosensorial equilibrium function measurements for special reprogramming and retraining purposes. In the field of diagnosis they place functional investigation of the equilibrium system alongside the other classical techniques which mostly work through inspection and imaging. Consequently, the MCS method of treatment (*m*echanics, *c*ybernetics, *s*ynergetics) has to take into account the basic knowledge on information transfer from the inner ear hair cells to the central nervous system in the regulating centers of the brainstem.

With this book an international group of neurootological investigators and clinicians describe in depth the clinical application of exercise therapy in the framework of a general neurootological treatment plan. Starting from theories for vestibular adaptive control mechanisms in patients with vestibular deficits and vertigo, and from vestibular tests which demonstrate the ability of reactional suppression and habituation, various kinds of physical and mental exercises were used to monitor and to stabilize the success of treatment in the long term. Combination of pharmacotherapy with treatment by physical and rehabilitation procedures was also taken into consideration.

The volume brings together a well-designed collection of the various basic and clinical experiments regarding the complex sense of the human equilibrium. As shown by the results published here, the MCS method represents a valuable addition to the therapeutic modalities of modern neurootology. It will be an aid both for medical doctors and those in related professions, especially physiotherapists, who are involved with dysequilibrium disorders.

Bad Kissingen, August 1998   Claus-F. Claussen

Contents

1 Introduction: Mechanics, Cybernetics and Synergetics of the Equilibrium System

Vertigo and dizziness are very common symptoms in the general population. Statistical research has found that, for example, they have a prevalence ranging from 5% to 10%, according to age class; they are particularly common in the population over 40 years of age, and they are the primary reason for a medical visit in many patients over 65 years of age.

There are no specific drugs for the treatment of these symptoms and there is no specific treatment for the most of the causes of vertigo and dizziness. Rehabilitation seems to be the most effective tool for the therapy of vertigo and dizziness. Although so-called vestibular rehabilitation, which is a special rehabilitation method for motion intolerance and imbalance problems, has only recently gained wide attention, the concept of head, body, and coordinated eye exercises as a treatment for vestibular disorders is actually over 50 years old. As far back as the mid-1940s, an English otolaryngologist, Sir Theodor Cawthorne, observed that some patients who experienced dizziness did better or recovered sooner when performing rapid head movements. In cooperation with a physiotherapist, F.S. Cooksey, he developed a regimen of exercises which, with some modifications, are frequently still used today. The Cawthorne-Cooksey protocol is based on the concepts of habituation and sensory substitution. These concepts are correct but they are not unique and they are perhaps not the best way of explaining the therapeutic effects of vestibular rehabilitation.

Vertigo and dizziness are conscious symptoms and the disturbances are not dysequilibrium or nystagmus but the *consciousness* of dysequilibrium and nystagmus. Thus physical rehabilitation must not only be targeted at resolution of the objective disorder but it must be aimed at resolution of the subjective consciousness of the disorder itself.

Such a specific kind of treatment needs a specific theoretical basis. For this reason we structured our method of rehabilitation on a particular model of the vestibular system.

The first consideration that led us to propose the following model was the need to think about a clear and satisfactory definition of "equilibrium." According to Massion, equilibrium control is correlated to postural control. Postural control is a behavior that involves "the maintenance of the alignment of body posture and the adoption of an appropriate vertical relationship between body segments to counteract the forces of gravity and allow the maintenance of an upright stance." According to Norrè, balance function "consists of a sensori-motor complex. The goal of this function is: stabilization of the visual field and maintenance of the erect standing position."

Neither of these two important concepts explain, in our opinion, the ultimate goal of this sensorimotor complex. Why is stabilization of the visual field or maintenance of the upright stance necessary? Why does balance "work in a subconscious way and under normal conditions a well-feeling is present rather than a detailed perception of every change"?

In our opinion the sensorimotor complex that controls balance, that we name the equilibrium system, is aimed at enabling the animal man to be a *man*, that is to say interacting with the environment, communicating with the environment and learning from the environment. "Into," "with," and "from" are the keys to understanding the reason why the vestibular system is so complicated and equilibrium is so important for animals in general, and for man in particular. "Into," "with," and "from" are the practical keys of the exercises we will propose.

Why have we named our rehabilitation protocols the MCS method? Because it is a model. MCS is the acronym of mechanics, cybernetics and synergetics. To prepare a particular protocol of treatment it is necessary to have in mind a particular model of the equilibrium system.

It is important to state the differences between model and theory. We do not want to present a new theory regarding the vestibular system but an innovative interpretative model of the equilibrium function. In fact, from an epistemological point of view, *theory* is a complex of logical arguments that are as valid as they are *true*. *Model* is a complex of logical arguments that are as valid as they are *useful*. In this way we prepared a model aimed at the treatment of vertigo and dizziness, using information based on modern neurophysiology theories of the vestibular system, movement control, cognitive processing and learning.

The basis of every complex function is a reflex. Thus for the equilibrium function, reflexes can be subdivided into two groups:

1. Ocular reflexes: vestibulo-ocular reflex (VOR), optokinetic reflexes (OKR) and cervico-ocular reflexes (COR). These reflexes make possible the stabilization of the visual field
2. Spinal reflexes: vestibulospinal reflexes (VSR), vestibulocollic reflexes (VCR), cervicocollic reflexes (CCR), cervicospinal reflexes (CSR) and stretch reflexes (SR). These reflexes make possible the maintenance of an upright stance and maintenance of postural control during moving (walking, stepping, jumping, etc.).

From a *mechanics* point of view we can consider the equilibrium function to be the result of the *sum* of these reflexes, the simultaneous but distinct activation of some or all of these reflexes, according to the need: gaze, standing or walking.

The neurophysiological organization of these reflexes is such that they are not always easily distinguishable from each other. Frequently peripheral information, such as visual or labyrinthine inputs, is conveyed on the same vestibular nuclei or the same reticular formation. Lackner stated that, under natural conditions, during movement, it is not possible to activate only single peripheral input. Thus Norrè proposed distinguishing two complex reflexes, each controlled by different sensorial inputs but generally elaborated in the vestibular nuclei and cerebellum: the balance ocular reflex (BOR) and the balance spinal reflex (BSR). The principle of this classification is the interaction between different sensorial inputs and different sites of elaboration.

From a *cybernetics* point of view all the structures, peripheral and central, that contribute to the BOR and BSR constitute a system. A system is a network of different *interconnected* structures, *interacting* to achieve a common goal. In this case the goal is human balance. The structures that provide the BOR and the BSR constitute the so-called equilibrium system. Lackner remembered that the so-called vestibular nuclei are real multisensorial relays and that they are not uniquely correlated to the activity of the vestibule. Thus it is incorrect to define those nuclei as vestibular nuclei. They are true balance nuclei that bring together cerebellar and reticular formations to provide the subcortical component of human equilibrium. From the neurophysiological point of view the equilibrium system (ES) is the vestibular system. In order to prevent any misinterpretation we prefer to refer to the equilibrium system as also including the vestibular part of information and reflexes.

A system is defined as any collection of components arranged and interconnected in a definite way, any collection of communicating materials and processes which together perform some function. From this point of view, labyrinths, eyes, vestibular nuclei, paravertebral receptors, antigravitary extensor muscles, plantar receptors, etc., constitute a system that performs the equilibrium function: the equilibrium system.

Systems are generally grouped into five main categories according to their different cybernetics aspects:

1. Lumped systems: the physical dimensions of the elements are very small compared to the wavelength of the input-output quantities. The system is distributed.
2. Time invariant systems and time varying systems: the system is time invariant if the elements of the system do not change their values with time; otherwise the system is time varying.
3. Linear systems: these must meet the homogeneity and superposition criteria, and the operators for input-output relations are independent of both input and output quantities. Other systems are "nonlinear."
4. Causal systems: a system which does not give any output unless an excitation is applied to its input is so defined. Otherwise a system is "noncausal":
5. Passive systems: in these systems all the elements are passive. If there are dependent or independent active elements or energy sources, the system is active.

The behavior of any system is determined by:
- The characteristics of the component or subsystems (e.g., threshold of stimulation of gamma-motoneurons, or endolymph characteristics)
- The structure of communication between components, which usually involves feedback paths (e.g., internuclear vestibular connections, cerebellovestibular inhibitory pathways)
- The input signals or variables to the systems initially assumed to be independent variables under the investigator's control

The ES, according to cybernetics, can be defined as a complex, open, causal, time-varying system. It is complex because it comprises different subsystems and it is controlled by different laws. The functional characteristics of the ES are the same as the complex systems in general and its rules are the same of those of the complex open systems: knowledge of these rules is the cornerstone of the therapeutic strategy for every type and site of lesion.

The ES is ruled by the following laws:

- Totality: every component of the system correlates with the other components. In this way a modification of one component has effects on the other parts and on the whole system: for example, a modification of the proprioceptive inputs may modify the vestibulo-ocular reflex and modification of the center of gravity may modify the activity of antigravitary lower limb muscles.
- Feedback: every open system is a circular system in which the outputs (eye movements, head movements, antigravitary contractions, etc.) of the system act as inputs themselves: muscle activity is itself a proprioceptive input to the system that controls the effectiveness of equilibrium output (so-called "reafference").
- Equifinality: in a circular self-regulated system the same functional effect can be obtained by means of action of different components or different arrangements of system components. This is the cybernetics basis for sensory substitution compensatory phenomena during the course of a vestibular lesion. Balance is maintained using different sensorimotor strategies in different persons and/or in different conditions. The same balance results are obtained both in normal subjects and in compensated vestibular patients when the interrelations between the different components of the system have been modified.
- Calibration: a system is steady if the components of the system remain within personally defined limits. This is the cybernetics explanation of the symptomatology threshold, which may be different between patients. From the cybernetics point of view we can state that, generally speaking, pharmacotherapy mainly acts to modify the calibration limits of the system.
- Preference: each ES is preferentially arranged in a precise and "personal" sensorimotor organization. Each subject maintains his antigravitary position using preferentially visual, vestibular, proprioceptive or somatoesthesic inputs. During rehabilitative treatment, exercises have to be planned following preferential sensorimotor strategies, if they are again effective for balance maintenance, or in order to modify sensorimotor preferential strategies if the "natural" conditions become (causing diseases) ineffective.
- Redundancy: the ES is based on redundant sensorial inputs (visual, proprioceptive, vestibular, somatoesthesic) and redundant motor programs (motor redundancy). Especially in aged patients symptoms are often due to a reduction in redundancy level both in sensorial and in motor aspects. Treatment needs to be aimed at increasing redundancy, and teaching the patient how to use residual sensorial information and how to optimize residual motor skills.

Cybernetics laws enable us to understand the complex organization of the ES but are again not sufficient also to cover cognitive aspects that, in human beings, underlie motor balance skills. Another model is thus necessary. When we treat a patients with vertigo or dizziness we have to keep in mind that they are human beings. That is to say that the patient presents consciousness of a disturbance of his or her ES. The disturbance itself and/or its consciousness prevents the patient performing what he or she wants: standing, moving, lying, moving the head, etc.

It is thus necessary to have in mind a model that interconnects the cognitive and movement aspects of human equilibrium. At the same time the model must lead to the simplification of the evaluation of the patient and the comprehension of such a complex system as the ES.

The brain, in fact, perceives sudden serial and intermodal integrated inner and outer stimuli and it programs coordinated reactions, physical and/or psychic. Perception ability is the functional basis of movement learning and it is sometimes more important than motor production skills. This is true especially for the particular motor skill named "equilibrium."

The *synergetics model* is based on the papers of Haken. He proposed his model to simplify complex functions such as macroeconomics processes, some physics phenomena such as cloud formation and many other complex phenomena. He proposed that every phenomenon, every function, is the macroscopic result of microscopic arrangements of the components that act together to produce the phenomenon itself (that is to perform the function). From this point of view a system can be subdivided into different functional levels. Each lower, microscopic, level communicates directly and is interconnected with the upper, macroscopic, level.

Equilibrium (which we can name E) is the macroscopic function. It is the result of the interaction of two main subfunctions: coordination and orientation. Coordination concerns outwards representation of the equilibrium while orientation concerns inwards representation.

The level coordination (which we can name EA) is the result of the interactions of lower functional levels:

- EAa: coordination of eye movements with head and body movements with respect to maintenance of continuous and distinct foveal vision
- EAb: coordination of tonic antigravitary muscle contraction and gravity force in order to maintain the desired position and shape of body (the so-called posture)

- EAc: coordination of tonic muscle contraction with gravity force and with dynamic phasic muscle contraction in order to obtain the desired movement (walking, jumping, running, etc.) into the environment.

The level orientation (which we can name EB) is the result of the interaction of lower functional levels:
- EBa: perception of the orientation of each part of the body with respect to each other part (perception of the body shape)
- EBb: perception of the orientation of the whole body with respect to the environment.

Vertigo and dizziness can be interpreted as the consciousness of an incorrect interaction between different functional levels of the equilibrium system. Thus, treatment planning must be aimed at reaching a correct and unconscious interaction between coordination and orientation, even if sometimes problems seem related only to a part of the function.

This book is subdivided into four chapters. In the first, the organization of the equilibrium system is shown according to the MCS model. It is not a true description of anatomophysiology. This is not the place to describe a detailed anatomy and physiology of the components of the equilibrium system. Rather we want to underline how the MCS concept enables us to build an anatomophysiological model of a system that represents the basis for diagnosis and treatment.

The second chapter of the book is dedicated to diagnosis. Also in this case it is not exhaustive regarding clinical and instrumental techniques, but it shows what it is possible to do clinically or by instrumental investigations in order to identify oculomotor, stance, gait and orientation involvement level of the disturbed equilibrium system of the patient.

The third chapter describes rehabilitative exercises. The protocols described need to considered as guidelines. In fact each treatment protocol must be strictly designed around the characteristics and the diagnostic findings of the specific patient.

Some of the exercises are not original and some of the instruments can be substituted with other similar ones. Otherwise it is important to emphasize that this chapter describes which physical and instrumental exercises are useful to deal with the mechanical and/or cybernetics and/or synergetics disorders of the equilibrium system of the patient.

Treatment is subdivided into different protocols specific for the most frequent situations that cause vertigo and dizziness. At the end of each part a paragraph is dedicated to how to maintain equilibrium by self-administered exercise, at home, after a period of rehabilitation performed with the therapist. It is important to underline that these exercises must be personalized and based on the personal program of treatment and they can never be substituted for the period with the therapist. In our experience if the patient is treated only by means of home protocols failure is certain.

Very common diseases such as Meniere's syndrome are not represented in this chapter. It is known that rehabilitation is not able to prevent vertigo attacks or to reduce progressive hearing loss. When the disease is stable, patients frequently complain of dizziness and unsteadiness even if acute attacks occur very infrequently. In this case patients can be treated with the protocol described under "Uncompensated unilateral vestibular hypofunction."

The aim of this book is not to outline a protocol for every vestibular disorder but to describe the guidelines of our rehabilitative method using some frequent imbalance problems as examples. It is important to underline that for each disorder, and specifically for each patient, a specific program needs to be planned and that this program should be based on the mechanics, cybernetics and synergetics aspects of the equilibrium system of the specific patient.

At the end of the book the "Bibliography" contains a list of papers and books that cover both neurophysiology and clinical applications. It is not a complete review of the literature dedicated to the vestibular system and vestibular rehabilitation and we apologize if we have omitted any important references.

2 MCS Organization of the Equilibrium System

Balance function aims to achieve a stable relationship between ourselves and the surrounding world, the environment. The result is spatial stabilization, which means that, when we perceive our surroundings, we have the impression that they are stable. During each movement of the body and/or of the head, the visual orientation of space has to be stabilized. The stationary objects which we observe in relation to our own position have to stay in the same place. This requires that, during movement, as well as when immobilized, the image of the perceived surroundings has to remain in the same place on the retina.

According to the MCS model, the equilibrium system can be interpreted as the result of mechanics components, cybernetics networks and synergetics functions. We can identify basic reflexes and simple motor outputs as mechanical components of the system, hypothesizing, in a simple manner, that each component acts independently of the others and that the functional result is the sum of different reflexes. These reflexes activate compensatory eye movements and compensatory antigravitational muscle contractions. In the first part of the chapter we describe the most important features of the reflexes on a "simple" ocular and postural movements basis.

2.1 Components of the System

Eye Movements

According to the traditional classification, eye movements can be subdivided into:
1. Voluntary eye movements that move the eyes in the desired direction
2. Automatic eye movements, provoked by a peripheral stimulation (generally visual) that maintains distinct vision of a target:

- Fixation movements
- Smooth pursuit eye movements
- Optokinetic nystagmus (OKN)
3. Reflex eye movements
   - Ocular movements that compensate displacements of the head in respect to the body
   - Ocular movements that compensate head displacements.

These groups of eye movements are controlled by different cerebral pathways:
1. The frontal cortex and the anterior pathways control voluntary movements
2. The parieto-occipital cortex and the posterior pathways control automatic movements
3. The brainstem and, particularly, the vestibular nuclei control reflex eye movements.

Another classification of eye movements subdivides them into only two groups regarding kinematics characteristics:
1. Vergence, disconjugate eye movements, that allows distinct foveal vision of a target when it is less than 20 cm from the eyes
2. Version, conjugate eye movements, to fixate, catch or pursue a target over 20 cm from the head. These are divided into two kinds of movements: (a) fast eye movements (FEMs) and (b) slow eye movements (SEMs).

Slow eye movements (SEMs) have low latency (120–150 ms) and low velocity (less than 80°/s). Generally they are used:
1. Following visual stimulation:
   - In smooth pursuit of a moving target
   - In the slow phase of the OKN.

The aim of this kind of SEM is maintenance of distinct vision of moving objects in a stable visual surrounding. Smooth pursuit movements compensate the retinal slip of the image with a continuous, slow movement of the eyes. They also act together with the vestibulo-ocular reflex in order to stabilize the image during head movement.
2. Following a labyrinth stimulation
   - In the slow phase of the vestibular nystagmus
3. Following a proprioceptive stimulation
   - In the slow phase of the cervico-ocular reflex.

SEMs depend on the afferent pathways which make up the extrageni-
culate system and the visual occipital cortex, associative parietal cortex and frontal oculomotor fields. The cerebellum is very important
in the control of SEMs. Particularly, the flocculus plays a fundamental
role in the gain of the vestibulo-ocular reflexes, allowing the stabilization of the image during head movement.

Fast eye movements (FEMs) are those movements that we usually
employ when we want to explore the environment. They have a long
latency (200–250 ms) and a high velocity, proportional to the width
of eye displacement (up to 800°/s). FEMs are used:

1. Following a visual stimulation
   - Catching a peripheral target or refixation of a target (e.g., during
     a lecture)
   - Pursuing a target the velocity of which is greater than SEM's
     range of action
   - Fixation adjustments with microsaccades
   - Fast phase of the optokinetic nystagmus
2. Rapid voluntary or automatic movement toward an imaginary target or a sound source
3. Returning of the eyes to the primary position after a slow deviation, such as nystagmus provoked by labyrinth or proprioceptive
   stimulation (fast phase of nystagmus).

Fast phases of nystagmus are controlled by brainstem structures
(pontine paramedian reticular formation) while automatic and voluntary saccades are principally controlled by frontal cortex.

Binocular vision requires perfect conjugation of the eyes, that is to
say a perfect equilibrium between agonist and antagonist ocular muscles. Conjugation of eye movements is performed by fibers running
along the medial longitudinal fasciculus (MLF) of both sites. Each
MLF correlates the lateral rectus of one site and the medial rectus of
the other site in order to perform contemporary abduction of one eye
and adduction of the contralateral eye. Recently a direct connection
between the paramedian pontine reticular formation (PPRF) and the
ipsilateral nucleus of the III cranial nerve has been demonstrated,
probably in order to support MLF (so-called para-MLF).

While the brainstem principally controls the latency of saccades
and basal ganglia regulate their velocity, the cerebellum is particularly
important in the control of the accuracy of saccades. This role is principally due to the vermis and fastigial nucleus. Lesions of these structures lead to dysmetric saccades. Flocculus is involved in the control
of the maintenance of the eccentric position of the eye when it is

moved. When it is lesioned, eyes, after an eccentric movement, slowly return to the primary position.

Foot

The foot is in contact with the supporting surface. In this way extero-ceptive information is included in the sensory input. The foot is an osteotendinous set particularly rich in neuromuscular Golgi spindles which are innervated by the orthosympathetic system. This system differs between races, which is why the arch of the foot differs between races: 125° in Caucasians, 145° in blacks and 135° in Asians. The shape of the foot is strictly dependent on the degree of tension of its intrinsic muscles, directly controlled by the orthosympathetic system. Extrinsic muscles are inserted on both foot bones and leg bones: the tibialis posterior, brevis peroneus lateralis, peroneus lateralis and flexor of the foot. Intrinsic muscles are inserted on the foot bones.

The sole of the foot is also rich in both superficial (Merkel and Meissner) and deep (Golgi-Mazzoni, Pacini-Water) pressoceptors. Information reaches especially the cerebellum either from the fuses or from the pressoceptors. The area of representation of the foot in the cerebellum cortex is wider than the area of the hand, exactly the inverse to the cortical cerebral representations. Proprioceptive and so-matoesthesic information reaches the vestibular nuclei through the cerebellum, which finely regulates the dynamic characteristics of the foot modifying the tension of the muscles.

Receptors of the foot are particularly involved in the regulation of the reciprocal spinal inhibition, termed 1A inhibition, which is one of the fundamental mechanisms of agonist/antagonist contraction regulation. In the cat the stimulation of the sole receptors facilitates the activity of spinal interneurons. In man, similar effects can also be obtained by stimulating the dorsal part of the foot. This seem to be correlate with the possibility of sudden corrections caused by unpredictable perturbations during a bipedal gait.

Vestibulospinal reflexes (from both canals and otoliths) are involved in the control of the activity of the 1A interneurons. Thus in the spinal cord there is the interconnection between vestibular and foot information, acting on the 1A interneurons.

Foot information projects to the Schwalbe, Roller, and X and Y nuclei through the reticular formation. At the same level somatoesthesic information from the skin arrives. These connections between skin, foot and labyrinth are necessary for a precise evaluation of the acceleration of the body during movement.

Ankle

The ankle and hip are two of the most important joints involved in maintenance of equilibrium during standing and walking. Even if receptors are present in all joints and tendons, these two joints seem to have particular concentrations of receptors. Joint receptors consist of:

1. A spray type or Ruffini endings located in the joint capsule
2. A larger spray type or Golgi endings located in the ligaments of the joint
3. Encapsulated paciniform endings commonly found in the fibrous periosteum near articular and ligament attachments. The discharge of joint receptors is related to the movement and position of the joint. These afferents project via the dorsal root into the lemniscal system, the thalamus and up to the cortex.

Sherrington (1947) postulated a contribution of joint receptors, and subsequent investigators believed them solely responsible for position perception. Recent electrophysiological studies have shown that joint receptors alone cannot give sufficient information to account for the accuracy of joint angle perception. Anesthetization of joints impairs kinesthesia only when accompanied by anesthetization of the overlying skin. Cutaneous receptors appear to support or facilitate the specific kinesthetic signals from intramuscular and possibly joint receptors. None of the receptors seem to be completely appropriate to the tasks demanded of them.

Perturbations of upright posture are corrected by viscoelastic forces inherent in the ankle muscles and provided ankle rotation is small (0.2°). In normal standing, ankle-foot proprioceptors appear to be more sensitive than vestibular proprioception. Normal persons, and trained persons in particular, can stand upright by making very small excursions controlled by proprioceptors. Experiments indicate that the pressure center is most sensitive to ankle rotation, less sensitive to hip rotation and least sensitive to rotation at the level of the shoulders. Most of the torque necessary to stabilize an upright stance is generated about the ankles. The importance of the ankle sensors is linked to the conception of the body as an inverted pendulum.

The reliability of the ankle-foot proprioceptive information is very much dependent on the nature of the support surface. Standing on a firm surface, angular acceleration velocity and position of the body are accurately reflected in the changes in the angles of the ankle and the pressure in the feet. On a stable support the anatomical angle of the ankle joint corresponds with the inertial angle.

When standing on a compliant surface or if the support is narrow or unsteady, the feet can move relative to the environment. Under these conditions reliable articular information is no longer available.

Antigravitational Muscles

Muscles can be subdivided into two groups: phasic and tonic muscles. Phasic muscles are characterized by the possibility of relaxation or contraction according to the need to produce a movement of a body segment. They are the muscles of movement. Tonic muscles are characterized by continuous "tonic" contraction of their fibers to maintain the position of the body segments. They are responsible for postural tone, which is a complex phenomenon mainly based on the activation of stretch reflexes. The main muscles involved in antigravitational action are the gastrocnemius, hamstrings, tibialis anterior, triceps surae and paravertebral muscles (Fig. 2.1).

The total number of afferent fibers to the muscles that act at a joint is large in comparison with the number of afferent fibers to the joint itself. A muscle spindle is a specialized form of muscle fiber, containing contractile elements as well as sensory endings. The muscle spindles lie in parallel with the extrafusal muscle fibers and receive their own motor innervation through small myelinated gamma efferents (fusimotor). There are two classes of sensory endings in the spindles. The primary endings are always present and are innervated by large-diameter, fast-conducting, low-threshold, group I afferents and are particularly sensitive to dynamic stretch. The secondary endings are innervated by smaller, higher threshold fibers and slow-conducting axons (group II). They are much less sensitive to dynamic stretch.

The receptors respond to changes in the length and tension of the spindle. When a muscle is stretched, the primary endings signal both the instantaneous length of the muscle and the rate of stretching, while the secondary endings signal mainly instantaneous length.

Each muscle spindle contains several contractile fibers (intrafusal fibers). The efferent fibers which supply the intrafusal fibers are known as gamma fibers. Efferent discharges in the gamma neurons cause the intrafusal fibers to contract. This stimulates the spindle sensory endings, which in turn affects contraction of the extrafusal muscles. In this way a complete feedback loop is established.

Golgi tendon organs are somewhat simpler sensory endings that lie in the musculotendinous junctions. Tendon organs respond to total tension in the muscle, whether this is produced by active contraction or passive stretch. They provoke monosynaptic inhibitory reflexes.

Fig. 2.1. Muscles involved in posture. *GCN,* muscle gastrocnemius; *HST,* hamstrings; *TA,* tibialis anterior; *TS,* muscle triceps surae

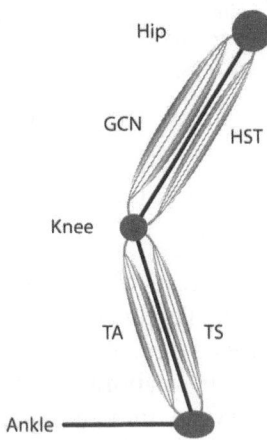

From a conventional point of view the stretch reflex is considered the main mechanism of postural activity. The basic reflex is the myotactic reflex (Fig. 2.2), which adjusts the muscular resistance to its elongation. Distension of the muscle stretches the parallel-coupled muscle spindles and activates the primary endings. These react to velocity change. The reflex arch of stretch reflex consists of muscle spindle, afferent primary and secondary fibers and efferent alpha motoneurons. The stretch reflex arch acts as a feedback system which allows the muscle to keep its length constant. This system is also active in the spinal postural muscles and enables the spine to keep upright. The effector of the stretch reflex, the alpha motor neuron, is influenced by:

1. Facilitating influences of the primary and secondary ending in the spindles
2. Inhibiting influences of the tendon afferences
3. Inhibiting influences by the intersegmental and supraspinal levels.

The stretch reflex occupies the key position in all conventional schemas, whereas the important role of other sources of afferentation is limited to information of descending influences that alter the reflex loop gain of the stretch reflexes.

Neck

The receptors of the cervical region play a separate and particular role and constitute what can be considered as a "secondary labyrinth." In a clinical context attention has been devoted to the neck

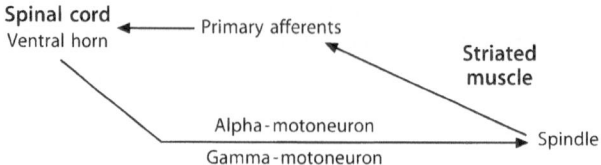

Fig. 2.2. Reflex arc at spinal level

with respect to a possible origin of vertigo, the so-called cervical vertigo. Furthermore its role in the posture of the head and the body seems undeniable. The cervical region with its structures intervenes in the elaboration of balance reflexes. Neck-body reflexes as well as cervical influences upon eye position have been described. It is the task of neck proprioceptors to inform the centers about movement or change of position of the head, so far as this concerns a differential movement between head and trunk. This is the fundamental difference from the vestibular system, which is sensitive to head movements relative to space. Both sensory systems provide specific and proper information, thus complementing one another.

Peripheral proprioceptors of the muscles and the joints have a feedback control of the vestibular nuclei through spinovestibular pathways. Neuromuscular spindles and Golgi receptors act as dynamometers and they are particularly sensitive to variations in muscle length and tension. Joint receptors and Ruffini and Golgi bodies give information regarding the position of a joint and its movement. The portion of the neck including the first three vertebrae is particularly involved during the major part of everyday head movements. The paravertebral muscles of this region are very rich in proprioceptors. They are especially concentrated in the m. splenius capitis, the m. rectus capitis major, the m. longissimus capitis and the m. semispinalis capitis. These muscles comprise the deep plane of the nuchal muscles. The splenius muscle is slightly more superficial. They act in the extension of homolateral bending and rotation of the head. During head movements they discharge to the vestibular nuclei.

Direct projection from the first three cervical roots to the inferior vestibular nucleus has been described, and the convergence of cervical and labyrinth inputs on vestibular nuclei has also been shown. Convergence especially includes inputs from the horizontal semicircular canal: the electrical stimulation of the vestibular nerve induces action potentials in the contralateral abducens nerve. This response is increased when neck roots are also simultaneously stimulated. Thus facilitatory convergences of proprioceptive inputs from C2–C3 receptors on the medial vestibular nucleus of the opposite side and an inhibition on the ipsilateral muscles have been demonstrated. The latency between electrical stimulation of the dorsal cervical roots and vestibular nucleus response is only 2 ms; thus direct projections from the neck to vestibular nuclei have been hypothesized. Proprioceptive nuchal afferences on the Schwalbe's nucleus have been demonstrated, and it has also been shown that neurons in the dorsocaudal portion of Deiters' nucleus receive tonic cervical inputs while the neurons in the rostroventralis portion especially receive otolithic inputs. Roller's nucleus and the accessory group Y receive ipsilateral projections from the cervical muscles, cerebellar projections on the nodulus and the flocculus have been demonstrated and projections on the cerebellar anterior lobus have been described. Proprioceptive convergences in 80% of the neurons in the suprasylvian parietal cortical vestibular area have been demonstrated and sensitive inputs run through IA and IIA fibers that rise along the spinal cord and through the spinoreticular and spinocerebellar fasciculus, which seem to send direct projections to the vestibular nuclei. Important evidence regarding the cervical control of balance comes from vibration experiments. The vibration of muscles or muscle tendons alters proprioceptive input and produces kinesthetic illusions in human subjects. Much clinical and experimental evidence exists regarding the effects of vibration of the paravertebral muscles on posture control and head-trunk coordination.

Generally the effects are based on the activation of the cervicospinal reflexes (CSR): bending the neck and turning the head relative to the body evokes reflexes in the limb muscles either in decerebrate cats or in human beings. These reflexes interact with vestibulospinal reflexes (VSR) controlling extensor muscle tone. Vestibular and proprioceptive inputs are integrated either in Deiters' vestibular nucleus or in reticular formation. Proprioceptive inputs are generated in muscle spindles of the neck muscles and they are partially responsible for the elicitation of CS reflexes.

The integration of the neck structures in balance performance is, however, more complex than a mere sensory contribution. The position of the head is governed by the neck muscles and the first guiding input is the vestibulocollic reflex (VCR). The cervical information by neck proprioceptors serves as feedback information. In this way a cervicocollic reflex (CCR) is generated.

The sensory input is produced by proprioceptors present in several tissues of the neck. The resulting reflexes are cervico-ocular reflex (COR) and CSR. The task of the neck muscles consists of stabilizing the position of the head relative to the trunk and of moving the head. This has to be executed each time to achieve the goal of balance, i.e., to stabilize the visual field and maintain the upright position. The neck muscles are controlled by the balance function via the VCR, which is a part of the VSR.

Lumbar Region

The lumbar region contains proprioceptor sensors similar to those of the cervical region. Galvanic labyrinthine stimulation with rotation of the trunk and the neck shows identical deviations. The lumbar captors are as important as the cervical ones in the regulation of posture. Lumbar proprioceptor influence has been shown in electromyographic (EMG) studies. Hypertonicity of the lumbar supporting tissues and especially the lumbar erector muscles is a cause of vertigo. Unilateral procainization of lumbar erector muscles causes swaying of the head, associated with unsteadiness of the body with drift reaction of the lower limbs often with ataxic features. There is a close correlation between changes in bodily equilibrium, such as the righting reflex and drift reactions of the lower limbs, and changes in cerebellar function. Lumbar proprioceptors are closely connected to the cerebellum through centripetal paths, such as the posterior spinocerebellar tract. In rabbits it was possible to elicit nystagmus by repeated unilateral electrical stimulation of the lumbar erector muscles, which was due to a functional disorder of the brainstem reticular formation brought about by repeated abnormal centripetal impulses from the proprioceptors of the lumbar erectors.

Vestibular Reflexes

During each movement of the head and/or body it is necessary that the image of the perceived surroundings has to remain on the same place on the retina. Thus the image of the perceived part of the environment must be changed very quickly. During head movement, the eye has to make movements relative to the skull in such a way as to guarantee immobilization of the image projection on the retina. If there is a "retinal slip," the vision is blurred, and the surroundings are perceived as moving around. As a result, during head movement the eye movement required has to be "compensatory," in order to cancel the effect of the head movement. Such eye movement is executed in a reflective manner, without conscious intervention, and it is called the vestibulo-ocular reflex (VOR).

The achievement of the correct erect standing position, under both static and dynamic conditions, requires continuous adaptation of the counterreaction of antigravitational muscles to the gravity force, in order to stabilize head position and to maintain the erect position itself. The maintenance of an upright position of the body is acquired via a continual to and fro movement of the center of gravity (CoG) around the point of mass equilibrium. This movement is called "postural sway." It is achieved in a reflective manner by the means of the VSR. The control of the correct head position is possible through the activation of the neck muscles by the means of a part of the VSR (the VCR) and the cervical reflexes.

On this basis it is obvious that vestibular receptors contained in the labyrinth must be of two kinds: one able to perceive movements of the head in order to activate compensatory eye movements (VOR) and one able to perceive the direction of the force of gravity in order to activate antigravitational muscles (VSR).

Semicircular canals (SCC) are the receptors whose function is to detect angular acceleration of the head and to activate compensatory eye movements. There are three of them, positioned in the three space planes. In humans the horizontal canals are inclined about 25–30° when the subject looks at the horizon but they are in the correct position during walking.

Otoliths are the receptors of gravity force and they furnish a constant inner basis of reference for both ocular and spinal movements. They are the main source of VSR. Otoliths are grouped into two orthogonal maculae, one placed in the utricle and one in the saccule.

Labyrinth receptors project to the vestibular nuclei in the brainstem, from which originate spinal and oculomotor efferent pathways through two reflex arches:

1. The direct arch is a trineural pathway the first neuron of which is in Scarpa's ganglion, the second one in the vestibular nuclei and the third in the ocular motor nuclei
2. The indirect arch trough reticular formation and cerebellum.

Vestibular nuclei can be subdivided into two groups: the main nuclei and the accessory groups. There are four main nuclei: superior, lateral, medial and descending nucleus. There are three accessory groups: X, Y and Z. Vestibular nuclei are real multisensory relays that integrate different sensorial inputs. Vestibular sensory integrations are part of the basis of the cybernetic organization of the equilibrium system.

The superior nucleus receives fibers from the canals and through the medial longitudinal fasciculus projects to the oculomotor nuclei. It also receives fibers from the vestibulocerebellum (flocculus, uvula, nodulus) and from medial and descending contralateral vestibular nuclei. It also projects to the cerebellum and the pontine reticular formation. It seems to correlate especially with the control of eye movements based on canal stimuli.

The lateral nucleus receives fibers from the utriculus and the cerebellum (vermis and tectal nuclei); a small part of fibers also arrive from contralateral vestibular nuclei and from spinocerebellar pathways. Efferent fibers constitute the ipsilateral lateral vestibulospinal pathway. A small part of fibers also reach oculomotor nuclei through ipsilateral and contralateral MLF. It seems principally to correlate with spinal reflexes.

The medial nucleus receives fibers from the SCC, maculae and cerebellum (tectal nuclei and flocculus). Minor fibers arrive from the contralateral vestibular nuclei and reticular formation. Efferent fibers make up the ipsilateral and contralateral medial vestibulospinal pathway. Some fibers also reach oculomotor nuclei, contralateral vestibular nuclei, the reticular formation and the cerebellum. This nucleus is involved in the control of eye, head, neck movements and vestibular compensation.

The descending nucleus (Deiters' nucleus) receives fibers from both SCC and maculae and from the vestibulocerebellum. It projects to the cerebellum, reticular formation and contralateral vestibular nuclei and seems to be involved in the integration of vestibular, cerebellar and reticular signals.

2.2 Cybernetics Functional Networks

The main characteristic of the vestibular nuclei is the integration of different sensorial inputs and control inputs (especially from the cerebellum). We explained how it is difficult to assign the single contribution of each reflex to a specific task, i.e., stabilization of visual images or stabilization of head position or upright posture. From the cybernetics point of view the organization of the equilibrium system has to be interpreted as the interaction of different subsystems. Each subsystem is made up of different receptors, different sites of signal integration and different sites of movement elaboration. It is not possible, under natural circumstances, during human movement, to recognize the contribution of each single component of each subsystem. Under every set of conditions subsystems have the function of controlling eye movements and of controlling antigravitational counterreactions.

Balance-Ocular Network

The first level of interaction between different oculomotor networks is represented by the *visuovestibular interaction*. For a long time it was difficult to recognize the anatomical pathways transmitting visual and vestibular information. Now, however, vestibular afferences to the visual system have been demonstrated; they pass through the superior colliculus and reach the visual cortex. Visual afferences also reach the vestibulocerebellum, especially the nodulus and the flocculus, and both cortical vestibular areas and vestibular nuclei: the vestibular neurons are thus activated either from the displacement of the visual field in one direction or from the displacement of the head in the opposite direction. Convergence of visual information on the vestibular neurons ameliorates sensitivity and neural responses during contemporary variation of visual and vestibular stimulations, especially when they are not congruent. This convergence allows either a correct ocular motor response during the movement of the head and/or the body, under natural circumstances, or a correct selection of the most appropriate sensorial information during constant stimulations. The ocular response provoked by simultaneous and congruent visual and vestibular stimulation is the so-called visuovestibular reflex (VVOR).

Visuovestibular connections have been well demonstrated regarding labyrinth stimulations. In the cat and the rat have also been demonstrated visuo-otolithic convergences aimed at the contemporary control of eye movements and posture. A convergence of visual inputs on vestibular nuclei pass through the cerebellum, especially the flocculus, by a polysynaptic pathway which includes the accessory optic tract and the inferior olive. There is another pathway for the pretectal nuclei, the prepositus hypoglossi nucleus and the reticular tegmenti pontis nucleus. Convergence of visual and otolithic information has the function of ameliorating the tachymetric function elaborating information regarding the velocity of the head, independently from the information concerning the acceleration and the frequency of head movements. Visual information is more important during slow movement frequency of the head and slow swaying of the body. Visual gain is higher than otolithic gain for frequencies lower than 0.25 Hz. At higher frequencies, the otolithic gain is higher than the visual one. Another role of the visuovestibular convergence is pursuit of a target combining both ocular and head movements. In this case, it is necessary to inhibit ocular movements provoked by labyrinthine stimulation. Thus, according to the cognitive task required, it is possible to optimize eye movements either optimizing the ocular motor gain (visuovestibular cooperation) or inhibiting vestibular inputs (visual inhibition). This use of the same gaze order (movement of the eyes and movement of the head) is typical of humans both when the subject moves the eyes only and when the subject moves eyes and head. The inhibition of the vestibular inputs by means of visual information is mainly controlled by the cerebellum and, secondarily, by associative parietal areas where neurons activated by visual fixation have been demonstrated.

A particular expression of the visuovestibular interaction is the *optokinetic nystagmus*. When the environment becomes wider than the visual field, vestibular and visual pathways cooperate in order to produce a complex eye movement constituted by a slow pursuit phase and a rapid resetting phase. It has been demonstrated that the integrity of the vestibular nuclei (and labyrinth) is necessary to produce a correct optokinetic nystagmus. It is now clear that generation of the optokinetic nystagmus is not a simple fast pursuit eye movement. It represents a primitive way to stabilize the visual field when the displacement of the environment is too large. The first part of the movement is phylogenetically ancient and is realized in the brainstem, involving principally the vestibular nuclei, being elicited by a stimulation of the peripheral retina. The second part of the optokinetic phenomenon is due to the stimulation of the foveal retina and involves the visual cortex and the pathways of smooth pursuit. This component provides the beginning of the movement, with velocities of the eyes up to 35–40°/s, while the vestibular component realizes the faster part of the movements with velocities up to 50–60°/s.

Passive rotation of the body is indicated by inputs from the semicircular canals and by the motion of stationary visual surroundings relative to the head. Vestibular inputs and inputs from visual motion detectors with large receptive fields converge onto cells in the vestibular nuclei and parietal cortex. When a person is rotated passively at a constant velocity with the eyes open, the response of the semicircular canals fades to zero over the first 30 s, leaving only the visual cue to self-rotation. In this initial period, the inputs from the two senses are averaged, but with an increasing weight given to the visual input as time passes. After vestibular inputs have faded, the only indication of self-motion is provided by the motion of the stationary visual surroundings relative to the head. It is as if the system knows not to expect a vestibular input after a period of constant rotation. When the body is stationary, motion of the whole visual scene, but after a while, as the weight assigned to visual inputs increases relative to the absent vestibular input, visual motion gives way to an illusion of self-motion known as circular vection. Thus vision extends sensations of self-rotation to low frequencies of rotation, including steady-state rotation.

VOR helps to stabilize the retinal image as we rotate the head. With eyes open the response is evoked by a weighted mean of inputs from the semicircular canals and inputs from motion detectors in the visual system. When the body is rotated passively in the dark about the vertical z-axis, the gain of VOR is inadequate at low frequencies of sinusoidal head rotation, but increases, sometimes to above 1, as the frequency of rotation is increased to 5 Hz. Visual inputs are more effective at low than high frequencies. When acting together, the two systems extend the frequency range of the VOR.

Man, in common with many other animals, has evolved a powerful system of hierarchical control mechanisms for stabilization of the foveal image, thereby ensuring maximal visual acuity. The afferent information necessary for effective control is derived primarily from the visual system and the vestibular apparatus, but also from proprioceptive information with special regard to that from the neck. The cervical contribution can be considered a "secondary" sensory input: the eye is moving in the orbit, while the ear is immobile in the petrous bone. For comparisons of the information from eye and ear, the position of the eye in the orbit has to be known. Here the oculomotor proprioceptors furnish a "secondary" input. With regard to summation effects of proprioceptions and vestibular inputs, the neck effect is most prominent with low-frequency stimulation in the horizontal plane, when the vestibulo-ocular reflex is poor. A comparison is made between active and passive attitude during sinusoidal head rotation in the range 0.05–0.33 Hz. Passive means that the head is fixed to the chair, while active means that the patient is instructed to stabilize the head with the trunk actively during rotation. The voluntarily stabilized head modulates VOR considerably. Saccadic activity and gain of slow-phase velocity are significantly enhanced as well as the amplitudes of maximum eye shifts. Moreover, phase relation is altered: in passive VOR the phases are around 180 and thus compensatory for body movement; in active VOR they tend towards 270, i.e., a phase lead of 90.

Vestibulocollic reflex (VCR) moves the head and interferes with the VOR for stabilizing the visual field. The VCR rotates the head in the plane of the canal. Natural canal stimulation results in contraction of neck muscles to counter the applied angular acceleration, and thus results in stabilization of the head. VCR augments the VOR for image stabilization during head movement. The *cervico-ocular reflex (COR) and cervicocollic reflex (CCR)* act to generate compensatory shifts of gaze which opposed those produced by rotation of the head. While the gain of COR is too small to make a significant contribution to gaze stability, the CCR is capable of generating large changes in neck muscle activity, which influences gaze and head position. In controlling gaze the VCR and CCR damp oscillations of the head and produce counterrotations that partially compensate for the rotation of the body, while the VOR compensates for residual rotation of the head with respect to space. In animals with vestibular lesions, COR and CCR increase to compensate partially. Head stabilization contributes to gaze stabilization.

Coupling of eye and head movement is a universal process. It occurs during voluntary visual orienting behavior as well as during reflexes that stabilize images on the retina. Movements of eye and head to an offset visual target consist of a saccadic jump of the eye to the target. This initial fast offset of the eyes in the direction of the object of interest is followed, after few milliseconds, by a head movement in the same direction. This results in an early target acquisition by the saccadic eye movement. Gaze direction is then held constant on target by a compensatory eye movement in the opposite direction of the head movement. This compensatory component is due to the VOR independent of any immediate corrective visual feedback. The gain of the movement is 1.0. Although the initial saccade was thought to be visually elicited, there have been recent suggestions that it may be generated by the VOR, its function being to contribute to target acquisition in the direction of the ongoing head movement. In monkeys, two modes of *eye-head coordination* have been described. The triggered mode is a response to an unexpected target. The saccadic eye movement occurs first (200 ms after stimulus presentation) and then after 20–30 ms delay the head begins to move in the same direction. Predictive movements occur after a period of repetitions and the monkey has learned to locate the target. The head begins to move well before (150–200 ms) the eye saccade.

When the head is rotated actively in the dark, the gain of the VOR remains at about 1 for all frequencies up to about 6 Hz, while it is lower when the whole body is passively rotated. This improvement in gain could be due to a potentiation of inputs from neck proprioceptors by active head movement or to efference copy associated with active head rotation. In either case, the improvement in VOR gain suggests that vestibular inputs and inputs indicating active head turning are weighted and averaged to produce a stronger stimuli than that produced by vestibular input alone. These results suggest that active head turning would produce nystagmic eye movements in the absence of vestibular inputs, especially at low frequencies of head turning where the gain of the VOR is low. Passive or active rotation of the trunk with head fixed induces a cervico-ocular response with a gain of about 0.2 at low frequencies of head rotation but hardly any response at frequencies above 0.44 Hz, and the response is often in a direction opposite to the VOR. However, the cervico-ocular response elicited by rotation of the torso with head fixed may not indicate the effectiveness of the response when it is elicited by rotation of the head. The absence of vestibular inputs in the head-fixed condition reduces the mean value of the combined inputs and indicates that eye movements are not called for. The cervico-ocular response is involved in more complex functions than that of supplementing VOR. For instance, it could be involved in the combined movements of eye and head when the gaze suddenly shifts to an eccentric visual target. In this role the two responses should cancel rather than complement each other since the eyes move in the direction of head rotation to acquire the target. The two reflexes (VOR and COR) also tend to cancel each other when the body is rotated with the head free to move.

Visuovestibular interactions involve not only the interaction between the version ocular motor subsystem but also the *vergence* subsystem. Stimulation of the vestibular system evokes the compensatory movements of VOR. The velocity of the compensatory eye movements required for image stability is zero for viewing at infinity because objects at infinity do not move detectably relative to the head when the head moves along a straight path. With the eyes open, any inadequacy in the linear VOR could be compensated for by OKN, which is naturally scaled for viewing distance because the angular velocity of the stationary scene relative to the head is inversely related to viewing distance. The scaling of linear VOR could be achieved in the dark if the response were coupled to the vergence state of the eyes. The gain of the VOR in the dark increases when subjects imagine that they are looking at a near rather than a far object. Linear VOR is inversely scaled for viewing distance as indicated by the state of vergence. Vergence provides the signals for modulation of the VOR, which are derived from the central motor command and are related to the shift of attention to the vergence target rather than proprioceptive feedback from the extraocular muscles.

Balance-Spinal Network

Three distinct sense organs respond to the sway of the body relative to a horizontal support surface: the vestibular canals and the utricle, the eyes and the pressure sensors in the feet together with the proprioceptors in the ankles and leg muscles. Posture is more stable when all the sensory systems operate. In the same way the direction of linear acceleration of the whole body is indicated by inputs from the otolith organs, by the pattern of optic flow of surrounding objects, and by proprioceptive inputs from the legs in active locomotion. Evaluations of direction and characteristics of linear movements may be made on the basis of any one of these cues, but are more precise and accurate when information from two or more cues is pooled.

However, inputs from the vestibular canals and somatosensory system stabilize static and dynamic posture more effectively at higher frequencies of body sway, while visual and otolith-organ signals are more effective at lower frequencies. The weighting of each cue is thus naturally adjusted by the frequency characteristics of each sense organ. The amplitude threshold for detection of body sway also differs between senses; the somatoesthesic senses have the lowest threshold, vision the next, and the vestibular system has the highest threshold.

Proprioceptors whose information reaches the vestibular nuclei are: the neuromuscular fuses, the tendinous organs of Golgi, the Pacini-Vater bodies and the joint receptors.

Afferent proprioceptive information is subdivided into the spinal cord, in two different parts: one lateral and smaller, the other medial with fibers with a larger diameter. According to their length they can be subdivided into short fibers, which reach the anterior spinocerebellar tract (crossed), medium fibers, which reach the posterior spinocerebellar tract (direct), and long fibers, which reach the gracilis and cuneatus nuclei in the medulla oblongata, and from there the thalamus along the medial lemniscus.

The most important pathways that control posture are the spinomedullothalamic pathway and the spinocervicothalamic pathway. Both are conveyed on the brainstem nuclei, before, and to the thalamus, after, different peripheral information from the muscles, the joint and the skin. Other fibers reach the olive, the reticular formations and the cerebellum. The fibers of the spinovestibular pathway input to the caudal parts of the medial, lateral and descending vestibular nuclei and the cellular group X.

Multisensorial convergence is especially important for the fine regulation of posture. Deiters' nucleus receives ipsilateral labyrinthine inputs and cutaneous, muscle and joint information especially from the lumbar region, and contralateral cervical information through direct (spinovestibular pathway) and indirect (spinocerebellovestibular, spinoreticulovestibular and spino-olivocerebellovestibular pathways). Schwalbe's, Roller's and the X and Y nuclei convey information both from the labyrinth and from the cervical region.

Cervical proprioceptive afferences are mainly crossed from the neuromuscular fuses of the paravertebral posterior muscles, which represent the extensor, tonic muscles of the cervical spine. Labyrinthine (from the vertical canal) and proprioceptive cervical information is conveyed on the spinal interneurons, mainly in the central cervical nucleus. From here, information reaches the cerebellum.

The interaction between vestibular and proprioceptive information modulates the vestibulospinal reflexes in order to stabilize the head and the arms with respect to the trunk, during the movement of the head in the space.

Stimulation of the neck induces different effects in man: it is able to facilitate or inhibit vestibular compensation after a lesion of the labyrinth (such as neurectomy) according to the site of stimulation, it is able to modify stabilometric body sway in normals, and it is able to alter the perception of the position of a visual target during eye-hand coordination tasks.

The cervical effect, however, has been proved to be somewhat dependent on the position of the head relative to the feet. With rotation of the neck alone, the direction of the sway varies directly with the neck rotation. With rotation of the trunk, with the neck stiff and the feet maintained in a fixed position, the sway is influenced in the same direction as with neck rotation. The sway direction is not changed, i.e., the face is kept in the forward direction while a trunk rotation is combined with neck rotation in the reverse direction. For any given head position in the horizontal plane, proprioceptive information from mechanoreceptors along the body is conveyed to equilibrium control centers providing information about the position of the head in relation to the support surface. Similarly to the cervical inputs, the foot input has the same "secondary" role in posture control: it has been related to the moving parts of the body such as the cervical and the lumbar spine.

The interaction between neck and labyrinth reflexes on the limbs stabilizes the position of the trunk with respect to the behavioral vertical. Interactions of the neck reflexes influence the supporting activity in the limbs related to the attitude of the head and the neck.

Labyrinth and neck reflexes produce opposite effects on the same limb extensor muscle. The tonic labyrinth reflex acts asymmetrically. Side down rotation of the head produces shortening, side-up rotation lengthening in the medial triceps. The tonic reflexes also act asymmetrically but in the opposite direction. This interaction of labyrinth and neck contributes to the stability of the trunk, allowing the head to move freely on the body without affecting stability. Neck reflexes are as important as labyrinth reflexes in the maintenance of postural equilibrium.

The interaction of vestibular and proprioceptive information involves not only the neck but the whole proprioceptive chain. When a person turns actively on a stationary surface, one would expect inputs from the semicircular canals and from the motor proprioceptive system of the legs to be averaged rather than summed because they provide independent sources of information about body rotation in the same inertial frame of reference. In other words, they constitute a multicue system requiring averaging, rather than a nested system requiring vector addition. This multicue system requires continuous reinterpretation. For example, motion of the ankle joint of a standing person can arise either from body sway or from standing on a sloping surface. A person standing on a horizontal platform moving to and fro in the dark maintains an upright posture by registering inputs from the vestibular system and from proprioceptors in the ankle joints and leg muscles. The two types of input covary and trigger a corrective contraction of leg muscles. A change in the angle of the ankle produced by concomitant rotation of the platform away from the horizontal does not conform to this covariance function. At first, subjects produce an inappropriate contraction of the leg muscles and their posture becomes unstable, but they soon reinterpret the proprioceptive inputs as signifying that the platform is both translating and rotating. We adopt this kind of cue reinterpretation when walking over an uneven surface.

Particularly important are also the proprioceptors of the oculomotor muscles. These are rich in neuromuscular fuses and of sensitive endings in the musculotendinous junctions. Primary fibers run together the motor fibers of the II, IV and VI oculomotor nerves, then they reach the Gasser nucleus through the ophthalmic branch of the trigeminal nerve. Some proprioceptive inputs from the oculomotor muscles also reach the cervical spinal cord, the mesencephalic reticular formation, the superior colliculus, the lateral geniculate body, the thalamus, the cerebellum, the vestibular nuclei and the oculomotor nuclei themselves.

Eye movements can influence posture without visual input. Eye position per se has influence upon posture and balance. An oculomotor-proprioceptive loop integrated in the total balance mechanism has been assumed. Vibration of the oculomotor muscles induces displacement of the body axis. Vibration of the superior recti muscle induces forward displacement, of the inferior recti muscle a backward shift. Vibration of the lateral rectus muscle of the right eye and of the medial rectus muscle of the left eye induces a leftward displacement and vice versa. Vibration of the inferior recti, sternocleidomastoideus or soleus muscles induces an analogous postural effect: a backward displacement. Costimulation of two of these muscle groups has a more powerful influence, but there is no dominance of one proprioceptive input over another. These vibrations result in an illusory perception of a slow apparent movement of the target in a specific direction. For a standing subject, the ground is the reference, providing the basic spatial information. The absolute eye-inspace position might be calculated by the CNS from the proprioceptive messages arising from the various body segments which link the eye with the ground.

The ability to maintain a desired static position (posture), standing, sitting or lying, without falling, is one of the most important features of the equilibrium system. This ability can be called postural stability and it is usually studied regarding a standing upright position. Maintaining postural stability involves coordination of mechanical components of the limbs, the trunk and the head and sensorimotor antigravitary network and it requires a correct perception either of the position of the whole body with respect to the environment or of the reciprocal position of each body segment The body movements used to the maintain postural stability are complex because of the number of joint systems and muscles involved. Sensing the position of the body relative to gravity and the basis of support is also complex and involves combinations of visual, vestibular and somatosensory inputs. Central adaptive processes are required to modify the sensory and motor components so that stability can be maintained under a wide variety of task conditions. The upright position can be expressed as position of the center of gravity (CoG) of the body regarding the relative positions of the whole body in the environment.

The center of gravity is the point at which the whole weight of a body may be considered to act. In humans who are standing quietly and vertically erect the CoG is located at the level of the hips and slightly forward of the ankle joints. CoG height is 0.5527 of total height. Center of gravity and center of mass (CoM) are equivalent points in space when the gravitational field is uniform and gravity is the only force under consideration.

When the body moves about the ankles as a rigid mass, vertically erect posture is observed when the CoG is directly over the center of feet support. In the anteroposterior direction, the center is halfway between the forward and backward boundaries of the support area. The body is vertically erect when the CoG is 14% of the foot length in front of the medial malleolus of the ankle joint. This alignment is equivalent to a baseline "forward lean" of the CoG of 2.3° with reference to an imaginary line passing through the ankle joints.

Maintenance of the CoG internal to the support surface perimeter requires a continuous control of the so-called postural tone. *Postural tone* is predominantly observed at the level of the limbs, back and neck extensor muscles, and the masseter muscle of the jaw. The main force vector of these muscles counteracts the effect of gravity when the subject is standing on a support surface. Postural tone depends on the integrity of the myotactic reflex loop and is suppressed by section of the dorsal roots. One possible mechanism for controlling erect posture is the stretch reflex, which would be able to oppose any deviation from the initial posture, but higher levels of control are involved. It is regulated by a series of reflexes which aim to maintain the reference posture or adapt it to changes in the position of the body segments. There are also three placing reactions: (1) the tactile placing reaction, in which the activation of cutaneous receptors on the soles of the feet causes activation of the extensor muscles of the leg; (2) the visual placing reaction; and (3) the labyrinthine placing reaction. The organization and the adaptation of antigravity postural tone mainly rely on spinal cord and brainstem circuitry. A tactile placing reaction needs the integrity of the motor cortex.

The functional role of the myotatic reflex in the leg extensors is limited to conditions of postural maintenance or slow precise movements. The mechanisms of the stretch reflex type play a minor role and are connected with preserving a particular pose. The major role seems to be played by the mechanisms carrying out the fast control of ankle and knee muscles through parameters describing the condition of general body equilibrium.

Stabilization of the head is a task of the neck muscles and is achieved by the integration of the vestibulocollic reflex and cervicocollic reflex. *Head stabilization*, in fact, also contributes to gaze stabilization as well as to the maintenance of the erect position. The head provides a stable platform for the elaboration of the otolith-spinal reflexes. Head stability is achieved by head movement mechanisms.

Head movement is a complex motor behavior that is controlled by more than 20 pairs of muscles that link the skull, spinal column and the shoulder girdle in a variety of configurations. The actions of these muscles are constrained by the physical properties of the vertebral column. Neck muscles are characteristically arranged in layered groupings. An outermost shell of long muscles connect the skull to the shoulder girdle. Beneath this outer shell a second set of layered muscles links the skull of the vertebral column. Most deeply is found a third set of muscles that closely invests and interlinks the vertebrae.

In all species the skull is commonly held at the top of a vertically orientated cervical column. In man the normal position of the head is that in which horizontal semicircular canals are parallel to the horizon. The head is then in the position characteristic of the usual attitude for reading, for examining something held in the hand or for walking over rough ground.

The cornerstone of stabilization of the head is activation of the vestibulocollic reflex. The VCR interacts with head-neck mechanical properties, voluntary movements and other reflex systems to determine the position of the head. The VCR activates neck muscles in such a manner as to counteract any head movement sensed by the vestibular system. The major function of the otolith-spinal projections to neck motoneurons is the long-term maintenance of normal head attitude relative to gravity. The stimulation of a single semicircular canal causes the head to move in the plane of the canal and in the direction opposite to the one which normally activates the canal. The plane of the head movement parallels that of the stimulated canal.

Movement of the head with respect to the body bends the neck and thus gives rise to changes in sensory discharge related to lengthening and shortening of neck muscles or deformation of tendons and ligaments. As for the other postural reflexes, the cervicocollic reflex is mediated in part by monosynaptic pathways in which sensory fibers synapse directly with neck motoneurons. Indeed the simplest spinal circuit is a monosynaptic pathway that links muscle afferents to motoneurons of the same muscles. In addition to the monosynaptic reflex connections, electrophysiological studies have revealed a long-loop pathway that could link neck afferent input to neck motoneurons. This involves neck afferents to the vestibular nuclei. Multisynaptic pathways also mediate cervicocollic reflexes through spinal, brainstem and cerebellar circuits.

Under normal conditions head movement provides a vestibular signal that gives rise to a vestibulocollic reflex acting to slow, or stop, the movement. In addition rotation of the head on the neck activates the cervicocollic reflex, which acts as a stretch reflex, as well as the optocollic reflex to oppose the applied disturbance. Dynamic properties and gains of the CCR and VCR are quite similar at frequencies between 0.2 and 3–4 Hz. VCR operates as a closed-loop negative feedback system: its output is the compensatory head position, which opposes and partly cancels the input driving signal.

Eye movement has been observed to precede neck movement, when preparing to move. This may interact with the neck reflex. In eye-head coordination a signal of "eye position" has to play an important feedback role for regulation of the interaction. This oculospinal loop has been called *optocollic response*. In several experiments, eye position-related activity in the neck muscles was found. Neck muscles show high tonic levels of activity relative to eye position when the head is fixed, whereas they usually discharge phasically in relation with head acceleration when the head is free. The patterns of neck muscle activation during eye-head gaze shift depend on the final gaze position. Each muscle has a preferential direction for which it is activated most strongly. Thus it could be shown that neck muscle activity faithfully reproduced eye position in head-fixed cats, where the EMG activity of a series of neck muscles was correlated with horizontal eye position. Not only does this muscular activity mimic spontaneous eye movements, but also eye movements during vestibular and OKN.

It is generally believed that the VCR is suppressed when subjects make voluntary head movements. The gain of the short latency is small and it is suppressed during active head movements, while the major control will be through longer-latency polysynaptic VCR, which is influenced by active head turns and is related to the direction of head movement.

Posture is controlled by otoliths but other graviceptive inputs have been demonstrated and they have been named *somatic graviceptors*. There are at least two separate graviceptive somatic inputs:

1. The first input enters the cord at the 11th thoracic dorsal root. Since at this point the renal nerve enters the cord, bilaterally nephrectomized subjects present the same postural behavior (in centrifugal experiments) of paraplegics. Experiments in bilateral nephrectomized patients have proved that kidneys contribute to gravity perception; however, it is an open question whether they function like statoliths or affect postural perception in another way, for example, by changing the parameters of the gravitational control systems.

2. The second input enters the brain cranial of the 6th cervical segment. Candidates for delivering information from the trunk to the

brain at a point higher than that are the n. vagus and the n. phrenicus. It has been presumed that the blood in the large vessels is the source of this kind of graviception. Its mass exerts inertial forces on the ligaments that support the vessel against the gravitational load. It presents the prerequisites for graviception: a density difference between the blood and the surrounding medium, and mechanoreceptors of the required type in the ligaments.

According to the hypothesis of "vascular graviception," the well-known fact that posture affects the vascular system is complemented by the reverse, namely, that the vascular system, via perception and control, affects posture too.

2.3 Synergetics Integrations

Strategies and Synergies: Basis for Motor Coordination

The ability to respond to perturbations to balance differing in direction, amplitude and velocity, during normal life activities, requires a complex organization that involves the brain control in regulating an incredible number of motions of the many mechanical linkages of the body and the activities of the associated muscle groups. It has been hypothesized that the CNS organizes movement in a hierarchical manner, with higher levels of the nervous system activating lower level *synergies*, which are groups of muscles constrained to act together as a unit. Bernstein hypothesized that breathing, walking and postural control would use synergies to coordinate the activation of muscles as a unit. Nashner and Woollacott demonstrated that responses activated in muscles of the leg and trunk in response to perturbations to balance are part of a pre-programmed synergic neural response and not the result of independent stretch and activation of individual muscles, due to a simple mechanical coupling of ankle and hip motion during perturbation. They showed how the movement of a single joint, the ankle joint, was able to activate the responses in multiple muscles.

The next step in the concept of the organization of equilibrium movements is the implementation of muscle pattern, or synergies, in strategies. *Strategy* is defined as the way which is selected to reach a goal. Regarding equilibrium, Nashner described two strategies that implement different muscular synergies in order to maintain balance during external perturbation: ankle and hip strategies. The same muscle pattern is associated with a given "strategy." When the external constraints change, the muscle synergy should change in order to achieve the same strategy. Strategy can remain invariant whereas the muscle synergies change, although the existence of fixed postural synergies when subjects are perturbed in the anterior/posterior direction has been demonstrated. When the center of body mass is perturbed forward or backward by displacing the support surface in the opposite direction, muscle activations begin in the ankle joint muscles and then radiate proximally in sequence to the thigh and lower trunk muscles on the same aspect of the body. This pattern is called the *ankle strategy* because it corrects sway by exerting torque against the support surface and rotating the body backward, primarily about the ankle joints. The ankle strategy uses torque about the ankle joints to resist gravity and rotate the body as a relatively rigid mass about the ankles. Constant ankle torques can be used to maintain offset center of gravity positions. Active ankle torques move the CoG over relatively large distances to a new position of equilibrium. Because the moment of inertia of the body about the ankles is large, only relatively slow CoG movements can be made using the ankle strategy.

When the subject stands on a support surface shorter than the feet are long, or when the CoG is located near the limits of stability, the same forward and backward displacements of the support surface activate the thigh and lower trunk muscles on the opposite aspect of the body. This pattern is called the *hip strategy*. It corrects sway by exerting a horizontal shear force against the support surface and rotating the body primarily about the hip joints. This strategy uses rapid rotational acceleration about the hips to generate transient horizontal shear forces. Because the moment of inertia of the trunk is small relative to that of the body about the ankles, the hip strategy can produce rapid forward and backward shifts in CoG position. The distances over which the CoG can be moved with this strategy are relatively small compared to those induced by ankle strategy.

Strategies represents the invariant aspect of the postural reactions related to equilibrium control, whereas the muscle synergies are partly fixed, partly flexible. Postural response synergies may be fine-tuned according to the task through learning and/or adaptive phenomena.

During voluntary movements particular strategies must be planned: *anticipatory postural adjustments*. In fact voluntary movement perturbs equilibrium for two reasons: the performance of a movement changes the body geometry and thus displaces the center of gravity position, resulting in equilibrium disturbance; the internal muscular

forces which are the origin of the movement are accompanied by reaction forces acting on the supporting body segments and will tend
to displace them. This will disturb both the position of these segments and equilibrium. Anticipatory postural adjustments serve together to control balance and to stabilize posture. Each type of anticipatory adjustment presents its own central organization and they are
under the control of cortical areas.

Movements of the legs are another source of disturbance of balance
because they take part in body support. The neural control by which
the center of gravity shifts toward a new position compatible with
equilibrium during movement is different from the neural control responsible for the anticipatory position adjustment, but it is highly dependent on motor cortical areas. A key aspect of balance during locomotion is the control of the mass of the head, arms and trunk with
respect to the hips. It has been hypothesized that the dynamic balance of the head, arms and trunk is controlled by the hip muscles,
with almost no involvement of the ankle muscles. Compensations for
balance perturbations during gait have been shown to be controlled
by responses in the ankle musculature.

Patients with functional balance problems are sometimes impaired
by lack of effective balance responses. The more usual problem is that
the patient's balance responses are inappropriate for the condition of
the task. Abnormalities in movement coordination can occur in three
forms:

1. The patient might select a movement strategy inappropriate for the
   task conditions and therefore appear uncoordinated. For example,
   small perturbations might elicit well-coordinated steps or stumbles
   rather than the appropriate ankle movements. Or the patient exposed to large perturbations might use a well-coordinated ankle
   movement and therefore fail to maintain stability. In the eye movement control system, the patient might use the vestibulo-ocular reflex inappropriately when the target he is attempting to track
   moves with him.
2. The patient might select the appropriate strategy, but the pattern of
   muscular contractions used to produce the selected pattern might
   be uncoordinated, leading to abnormal (rather than inappropriate)
   movement pattern. In executing an ankle movement, for example,
   the knee joints might buckle, because the thigh muscles contract at
   the wrong time.
3. The appropriate movement strategy might be selected and coordinated, but the movement onset might be delayed (latency), or the
   movement amplitude might be too strong or weak in proportion to

the stimulus (amplitude scaling). In the eye movement control system, for example, a saccadic eye movement to a target might overshoot.

Brainstem and Cerebellum: Who Is the Teacher and Who Is the Pupil?

Cerebellum and brainstem circuits are essential for the development and expression of the most basic form of associative learning. Normal human movements performed under equilibrium conditions can be considered to be harmonic with a continuous interconnected coordination and orientation. These interconnected "movements," in each instant, are also based on a psychological and attentive subject mental set (so-called cognitive aspects of "equilibrium") and they are regulated on the basis of visual, vestibular, auditory and proprioceptive feedbacks.

If we consider normal human equilibrium as the result of an interactive, associative and unconscious learning over years, we can also interpret equilibrium disorders as the results of disadaptive, nonassociative, sensorimotor uncoordinated and unfinalized movements. Nystagmus itself has to be considered a disadaptive and unfinalized movement of the eyes. One of the most important functions of the whole brain and especially of the cerebellum is, in fact, the ability to inhibit uncoordinated and unfinalized motor activities and simultaneously to facilitate those functions that allow human physical and psychic perception. The selective ability of nonuseful activity inhibition and useful activity facilitation is one of the functional bases of the so-called "plasticity" of the brain.

The two principal inputs to the cerebellum are climbing and mossy fibers. Climbing fibers come entirely from the neurons of a structure in the brainstem termed the "inferior olive." The climbing fibers send collaterals to the deep nuclei and project to the cerebellar cortex, where a given Purkinje cell receives a powerful excitatory synaptic input from one, and only one, climbing fiber.

The inferior olive receives its primary sensory input from the somatic sensory systems (skin, joints, pain, etc.), but it is also connected to other sensory circuits.

The mossy fibers originate predominantly from neurons in the pontine nuclei of the brainstem, but from other sources as well, for example, direct somatic sensory input. They project to the cerebellar cortex, where they synapse on granule cells. Mossy fibers also send collaterals to the deep nuclei.

The granule cells project to the Purkinje cells as parallel fibers. A given parallel fiber contacts hundreds of Purkinje cells with excitatory synapses. The pontine nuclei receive projections from many places in the brain, including heavy projections from the cerebral cortex. In terms of input to the cerebellar cortex, the climbing and mossy-parallel fiber systems are thus quite differently organized. The responses of a Purkinje cell to mossy-parallel fiber activation and climbing fiber activation are quite different. Thus, the activation by parallel fibers yields single action potentials, termed "simple spikes." The spontaneous rate of activation of Purkinje cells by granule cells (parallel fibers) is quite variable and can range as high 50/s or more. Activation of a Purkinje cell by a climbing fiber yields a very brief, for only a few spikes, later spikes in the train (several hundred per second) that last for only a few spikes. This Purkinje cell response to activation by a climbing fiber is termed "complex spike." The simple spike response to parallel fiber activation and the complex spike response to climbing fiber activation are easily distinguished in extracellular single unit recording from a Purkinje cell.

There are several types of inhibitory interneurons in cerebellar cortex such as Golgi cells, stellate cells and basket cells. Indeed the only excitatory neurons in cerebellar cortex are the granule cells giving rise to the parallel fibers. All other neurons in cerebellar cortex are inhibitory and are thought to use gamma-aminobutyric acid (GABA) as their inhibitory neurotransmitter. The Golgi neurons are activated primarily by parallel fibers that then make inhibitory synapses on granule cells, thereby constituting an inhibitory feedback loop. The stellate and basket cells are activated by the parallel fibers and exert inhibition on the Purkinje cells (feedforward inhibition).

The only output from the cerebellum comes from the cerebellar deep nuclei, which project both to the higher brain structure and to lower brain structures (interpositus nucleus of hypoglossi). Purkinje cells are the only neurons that project information out from the cerebellar cortex and they project only to the deep nuclei. Furthermore, their synaptic actions are thought to be entirely inhibitory.

Like the cerebral cortex, there are several different regions of cerebellar cortex that contain representations or maps of the body; information about events of the skin of the body are represented in multiple redundancy. But unlike those in cerebral cortex, these maps do not have topological "coherence." In cerebellar cortex the representation of various regions of the body appears to be chaotic (e.g., eyelid region next to the finger region). This incoherent mapping has been termed "fractured somatotopy."

The climbing fibers have very localized and powerfully excitatory actions on the Purkinje cells. This organization led theorists to the notion that the localized climbing fiber input acts on cerebellar cortex as the teaching input while the distributed mossy-parallel fiber input acts as the learning input.

Using mutatis mutandis classical theoretical and modern computational models we can attribute to the cerebellum a major role in motor learning and in equilibrium teaching.

The main functional differences between equilibrium disorders in cerebellum injuries versus brainstem injuries are essentially based on these distinctions:

1. Brainstem contributes to movement and equilibrium, informing the cerebellum and providing to the cerebellum learning information.
2. Cerebellum learns through sensorial and proprioceptive feedback (via the brainstem) and teaches the brainstem how to learn, regulating, in this way, movements and equilibrium.

An experimental set aiming to evaluate the role of the cerebellum in motor (and equilibrium) "teaching" is the evaluation of adaptive behavior of the vestibulo-ocular reflex (VOR) to the changing conditions brought about naturally by cell loss, disease, and aging, or artificially in the laboratory by prism glasses that alter the visual field.

The ability of the cerebellum to detect and repair this "dysmetria" that would otherwise cause motor incoordination indicates that more than a simple open loop control system is involved; feedback as to the accuracy of the eye movements is clearly being provided to the cerebellum by the visual system. Thus a slip of the retinal image signals the cerebellum to recalibrate the VOR. This recalibration signal must indicate the exact nature of the necessary change in the VOR, for example, how much of an increase or decrease in the gain will correctly recalibrate the reflex.

The vestibulocerebellum is the main instigator of VOR adaptive behavior. It can be defined as the "flocculi, the ventral parafloccull, the lateral third of dorsal paraflocculi, the nodulus, the uvula, the lower half of lobe VIII, and the lower three or four lobules of the paramedian lobules." The vestibulocerebellum is critical in the maintenance of the VOR. After vestibulocerebellar lesions, the VOR remained unchangeable no matter what was done to them. The vestibulocerebellum is necessary to produce and maintain the large plastic changes that are observed in the VOR when it must adapt to changes in the visual field.

The flocculus region of the vestibulocerebellum is critical for adaptation. The primary vestibular fibers project to the flocculus as mossy fibers. The flocculus also receives climbing fibers from the retina that contain error information about retinal slip: the discrepancy between the image that ought to project to the fovea and the "erroneous" image that does project to the fovea. It should be noted that the precise locus or loci of neuronal plasticity that codes adaptation of the VOR is still a matter of discussion, but authors agree that the cerebellar cortex of the flocculus is necessary for adaptation of the VOR and there is experimental evidence of memory trace location either in cerebellar cortex or in interpositus nucleus. The medial vestibular nucleus participates in cerebellar control of VOR adaptation and, in fact, it can be considered a deep cerebellar nucleus, displaced to the brainstem, in terms of its connections, for example, monosynaptic projection of Purkinje cell axons.

An "adaptive filter" model of the cerebellum to formally account for the adaptive abilities of the VOR has been proposed. While modulating the VOR, Purkinje cells are presumed to receive sinusoidal input of various phases from the mossy fibers via the granule cells and parallel fibers. Within this model the Purkinje cells learn to respond selectively to the various phase versions until they only respond to a very specific combination of inputs; that is to say, they adjust the synaptic weights on the parallel fiber inputs so that when summed at the Purkinje cell, the desired output is produced. In Fujita's adaptive filter model, Purkinje cells are presumed to perform a filtering function on the basis of multiple pairs of input signals and corresponding desired output signals. The Golgi cells are postulated to work at phase lag elements that act as a leaky integrator with a time constant of a few seconds. The output from this network, that is, the parallel fiber signals, would then represent different versions of compensators at different phase lags, depending on the relative weights of the inputs. The outputs of the parallel fiber signals are gathered together through various synaptic connections, which possess modifiable weights, to form the desired Purkinje cell output, that is, the final signal. The weights assigned to the individual parallel fiber signals are adaptive and plastic. They are adjustable depending on the desired output and how close the actual output of the Purkinje cells is to this desired output. The climbing fiber afferent inputs into the cerebellum which originate in the inferior olive and form powerful excitatory synapses with the Purkinje cells are presumed to be responsible for the learning capabilities of the adaptive filter. In other words, the mossy fiber afferents carry information to be processed by the cerebellum and the climbing fiber afferents carry a "teaching signal" to the Purkinje cells. The activity of the climbing filter inputs is determined by the discrepancy between the actual and the desired Purkinje cell output relative to its spontaneous discharge rate.

A close parallel can be drawn between the error signaling role of the climbing fibers in adaptation of the VOR and the reinforcing or teaching role of the climbing fibers in classical conditioning Pavlovian experiments.

Two quite different behavioral forms of learning, classical conditioning of discrete behavioral responses and adaptation of the VOR, have converged quite remarkably toward a common neural substrate. The cerebellum and its associated brainstem circuitry are necessary and sufficient for both forms of behavioral plasticity. In both paradigms a key event is a depression in the frequency of firing of Purkinje cells as a result of training or adaptation. A decrease in Purkinje cell firing will yield an increased neuronal response in interpositus (classical conditioning) or in vestibular nuclei (VOR adaptation), which increases the probability of a behavior response.

The characteristics of equilibrium disorders in brainstem and/or cerebellar diseases and their possible treatments are dependent on the different interactions between learning and teaching. In other words we can state that the brainstem teaches the cerebellum how to learn what cerebellum itself has to teach the brainstem. That is to say that in the brainstem inputs and outputs run in parallel while in the cerebellum these two signals cross and interconnect and large disruptions can be caused by small lesions.

The scope for treatment is based entirely on the residual capability of brainstem learning and cerebellum teaching. Using this kind of model it is easy to understand that the dysfunction will be worse and the treatment possibilities will be reduced if the injury is to the teacher (cerebellum) while the therapeutic results will be potentially better if the injury is to the learner (brainstem).

Internal Representation of Posture and Orientation

One of the main tasks in motor control is to orient the body with respect to the external world. This orientation is necessary for the appropriate coding of the information collected by the sensory organs on the state of the environment. In this respect, the orientation of individual segments, and especially of head and trunk, is critical.

Body orientation is under multimodal control and influence. In virtually any terrestrial circumstances involving natural movements, changes in peripheral vestibular activity will be accompanied by changes in the activity of somatosensory, proprioceptive, visual and auditory receptors. Consequently, it is difficult to ferret out a specifically vestibular contribution to orientation. In fact, it may not be possible, even in principle, to identify a solely "vestibular" contribution because of the convergence of vestibular, visual, auditory, somatosensory and proprioceptive signals in the vestibular nuclei.

The sensory information provided by visual, vestibular, proprioceptive and somatoesthesic inputs composes a complex image, which represents a typical pattern for each particular situation perceived. To constitute this pattern, the primary signals from the sensory organs are transduced to a more suitable signal, whereas selective utilization of these signals contributes to the adequacy of the final signal.

Balance function is developed progressively by experience. Patterns, processed previously, constitute a stock of reference patterns. This means that many situations can be processed in a normal, unconscious way. The incoming pattern has to be harmonious, each sensorial input furnishing information which is not contradictory to that of the other.

Bodies of terrestrial creatures are dynamically adapted to the 1-g force background of Earth. In a certain sense, this is obvious. Creatures on Earth are adapted to the terrestrial force of gravity background acceleration level. The nature of these adaptations is especially important because we are not normally aware of their existence. For example, consider what we experience under terrestrial conditions when we shift our stance from two feet to one, namely, a small change in force on the standing foot, a slight increase, if any. Yet the force on the standing foot has doubled. The failure to perceive the force increase is actually part of our dynamic adaptation to Earth's gravity such that near constant levels of force are experienced on the feet during voluntary stance and locomotion. When running, for example, the forces on our feet vary from 0 to 3 times of our body weight; yet this enormous fluctuation is not perceived.

Individuals regulate the position of the center of gravity with respect to the ground through the use of a postural body schema, which includes an internal representation of vertical, of body kinematics and of body kinetics. The main substrate as the basis for body orientation is the so-called *postural body schema*. This internal representation of body posture has been hypothesized to be partly genetically determined and partly acquired by learning and to include the main aspects of vertical geometry and kinetics.

Sensory information providing orientation inputs is combined in a great variety of ways for diverse purposes. It may be combined from different receptors or different feature-detection systems within a sensory system (intrasensory interaction) or from distinct sensory systems (intersensory interaction). There are also interactions between the corollary discharge accompanying motor commands and sensory input (reafference) arising from the motor activity. Sensory interactions can be interpreted as different models. For example, to judge the position of one hand, orientation information providing inner reference is organized according to a nested model. A nested sensory system consists of sense organs embedded in series, or a chain, of jointed body parts. A nested task is one that depends on inputs from two or more nested sense organs. The sense organs belong to the same sensory modality. For example, inputs from proprioceptors (joint receptors, tendon receptors and muscle spindles) associated with the shoulder, elbow and wrist form an intersensory nested system with which we perform the nested task of judging the position of an unseen finger relative to the trunk. The efference copy associated with active movement at each joint can also be regarded as a sensory input. The lengths of limb segments are not provided by either sensory inputs or motor efference, but are learned during visually guided teaching, and they change as the body grows. They form an essential part of the body schema, or internal representation of the body. Another aspect of the body schema is that we know the positions of body landmarks, such as the nose and the navel, even though the somatoesthetic senses serving them may be anesthetized. The incredibly rich and detailed knowledge that we have about our bodies operates largely at a preconscious level and is involved in every action that we carry out. A nested system of joints, such as the arm or leg joints, allows us to perceive the direction, motion or distance of an object within reach of the limb. Nested organization of sense organs is used for judging the position or motion of one part of the body relative to another part of the body or with respect to gravity or a contact surface. It can also be used to coordinate the motions of the arms or legs, which contribute to the control of body posture and to stabilization of the head, eyes, and retinal image in space. In the motion domain, there are mechanisms that extract the relative velocity and direction of motion of two objects. These mechanisms form the basis for the visual recognition of complex patterns of relative motion such as the motions of the parts of the human body. The nested set of proprioceptors in the wrist, elbow and shoulder locate the hand with respect to the torso, and the retina-eye-head system locates the light with respect to the torso. The neural coordinate systems used to register each component must be transformed into a common form. Even

without practice, one can point to a visual target with an unseen finger with a precision of about 2°, although people tend to overshoot
the target when it is presented in an eccentric retinal location. Both
visual and proprioceptive information about initial arm position are
used in planning an arm movement.

The individual's geometric representation of the body mainly depends on the information provided by the proprioceptive Ia afferent
inputs. Proprioception from all parts of the body plays an important
role in the maintenance of quiet stance body posture. When an individual is standing, there is a kinematics chain formed by the Ia inputs from muscles around each joint, informing the central nervous
system (CNS) about the position of each joint with respect to the remaining parts of the body. The output of the spindle primary fibers
is interpreted differently by the CNS depending on such factors as the
selected reference frame of the subject (the body as reference frame
or three-dimensional environmental coordinates) and the presence of
gravity. Proprioceptive Ia afferent inputs monitor both body displacement and velocity of displacement. Postural response to labyrinth
stimulation depends on the head position with respect to the trunk
and the head-trunk position with respect to the legs.

The postural control does not behave as a single functional unit. It
reveals an organization into "modules," superimposed from the feet to
the head. Each module is tied to the next one by a set of muscles
which have their own central and peripheral control, aimed at maintaining the reference position of the module. The modular organization can be modified according to the task by changing the joint stiffness of one or several joints in order to build up new modules. The
modular organization of posture can serve to regulate posture itself.
The stabilization of the head in space during locomotion is used as a
navigational inertial platform for the evaluation of the visual or labyrinthine inputs signaling changes of body position with respect to the
external world. Modular organization serves as an egocentric reference frame for the organization of movement. For example, during a
teaching task, head and trunk axes are a reference value for the calculation of the target position with respect to the body and for calculation of the hand trajectory. During manipulation of heavy objects, the
forearm position is stabilized and serves as a reference frame for this
task.

Two aspects concerning body kinetics should be mentioned: the
nervous system's evaluation of the support conditions and the calculation of the inertia of different body segments, used for providing an
accurate estimation of the center of gravity position. During stance,

reaction forces are exerted by the supporting platform of the body. They are the main basis for the maintenance of the erect posture. It is generally admitted that stance results from a support surface oriented maintenance of balance, on the basis of these reaction forces. The foot sole receptors and proprioceptive inputs from foot muscles play a role in perceiving the reaction forces. There is an internal representation of the support conditions, which selects the appropriate actuators for optimizing the equilibrium maintenance. In fact when the body weight is reduced, such as in water, the postural reactions tend to disappear. A second aspect of body kinetics is the inertial properties of the segments and their mass. These properties are automatically taken into account for the regulation of balance.

The *orientation of body* with respect to vertical in the frontal plane and in the sagittal plane is a primary constraint for erect posture in a world in which the effects of gravity must be taken into account. There are no static sensors which directly monitor the center of gravity projection to the ground. The body orientation with respect to vertical in the frontal and sagittal plane is regulated by both sensors located in the head and in other body segments. The sources of information regarding orientation with respect to verticality are the otoliths, the visual static inputs as the vertical and horizontal structure of the visual frame (the objects within the visual field), and the so-called somatic graviceptors.

Looking at an environment that is coupled to the head movements gives erroneous visual information, because during the stance body sway is not correctly sensed. In this condition the subject tends to orient posture to the orientationally incorrect visual vertical reference. A sensory reference is selected which fails to signal changes correctly in orientation to Earth's vertical during body sway. Whereas complete loss of vision only minimally affects equilibrium, visual distortion can have a significant effect on balance. The influence of this kind of distortion can be evaluated fixing an internally illuminated box around the subject's head in order to stabilize vision with respect to head/body movements. It could be shown that eye closure provokes a weaker amplitude of body sway after rapid perturbation than stabilization of the vision by the box. Another way to show the importance of visual distortion in the control of orientation is the tilting room that provides an erroneous visual vertical.

Experiments provide evidence in favor of the assumption that sustained activity of eye muscles can influence the equilibrium of the body. Vision may have a strong destabilizing effect on posture, especially when visually perceived motion does not adequately correspond to the actual body shift sensed by vestibular and somatosensory systems.

Understanding the correlation between vestibular responses and perception is of key importance for understanding the etiological bases of vertigo and dizziness.

Of interest are the experiments performed during weightlessness and during parabolic flights. In these experiments VOR, perception of body orientation and symptoms were studied during exposure to Coriolis cross-coupling stimulations. Such stimulation occurs when an individual who is rotating tilts his head out of the axis of rotation. This leads to an atypical pattern of activation of the semicircular canals and otolithic maculae and can be profoundly evocative of motion sickness and disorientation. The results of experiments indicate that immediately on transition to free fall, a condition near to weightlessness, Coriolis cross-coupling stimulation is much less provocative and disorienting than in straight-and-level flight (1 g, normal gravity force exposure). By contrast, exposure to 1.8 g (near to twice the terrestrial gravity force), a much greater than normal background force, produces immediate and dramatic increases in provocativeness and disorientation. Curiously, however, the VOR are not influenced as strikingly. The step gain of the VOR to cross-coupling is not affected by different background force levels. This means that the peripheral response of the semicircular canals is not affected by background force level.

Observations during weightlessness and parabolic flight regarding perception of orientation of the body may relate to the discovery of "place cells" in the hippocampus of experimental animals. Such cells are active when the animal is in particular locations in a familiar environment. They also seem to be modality independent in terms of their excitation; for example, vision is not necessary to activate them. Episodes of "nonorientation" in a weightless environment raise the possibility that otolithic and/or touch-pressure activity may be necessary for place cells to be functionally activated, at least during initial exposure to weightlessness. Such exposure imposes the need for wide-ranging sensorimotor recalibrations that affect the control of the head and the body, as well as strategies for orientation and movement activities. Alteration in vestibular function is an important concomitant of exposure to weightlessness and the need for adaptive accommodation but is not the sole factor contributing to disorientation and space motion sickness. The changes in body weight that occur in a non-1-g force environment also affect movement control and contribute to motion sickness.

Experiments in weightlessness emphasize the importance of integration of multisensorial information to correct orientation perception of the head and the body in the environment. These experiments lead to the interpretation of vertigo and dizziness also as a consequence of central misinterpretation of peripheral signals and/or erroneous interpretation of signal integrations. This is particularly important in the interpretation of dizziness, in which the disorientation symptomatology component is predominant.

During a normal stance, graviceptors monitor the force vector exerted at each joint to oppose gravity and this information contributes to an internal representation of the vertical axis. A putative candidate for the monitoring of this sensory information is the Golgi tendon organ, which measures the number of active motor units at a given time in each muscle used in the postural control. In addition the stabilization of balance by body sensors depends mainly on muscle Ia afferent proprioceptive input, which indicates any changes in the position of one segment with respect to its neighbors and, as a result, induces postural adjustments.

An important role is played by cutaneous foot sole sensors and foot muscle proprioceptors, which monitor the amplitude and the direction of the contact forces exerted by the body onto the ground.

Sensory organization of proprioception and exteroception is fundamental for the orientation of the subject into the environment. Intersensory comparisons of different inputs allow the growing child to form associations between the sounds, visual features, tactile properties and smell of objects. They also provide the basis for the development and maintenance of a consistent internalized spatial metric (the inself) that have to be continuously compared with information regarding the environment (the outself) in order to provide location, directions and distance of visual landmarks, sounds and odors helping animals, in general, and human beings, in particular, to navigate. The effectiveness of a movement performed for navigation or to reach an object also depends on the effectiveness of the stimulation of the sense organs produced by movement itself. This feedback information has been defined "reafference," to distinguish it from exafference, which does not arise from voluntary movement. Efference copy scaled by reafference expresses the invariant relationship between voluntary motor commands and consequent sensory stimulation. Over many repetitions of voluntary movement, the subject learns how efference and reafference are related. A mismatch between current efference and proprioceptive reafference and the learned pattern signifies that some of the efference is used to overcome or restrain an externally applied force. A mismatch of exteroceptive reafference signifies that part of the signal is due to external events. A persistent mismatch in either type of reafference, proprioceptive and exteroceptive, signifies that the system is in need of recalibration. This happens as the body grows during infancy or when the system is disturbed by injury.

3 Evaluation of the Patient Suffering Vertigo and Dizziness

The patient suffering vertigo and/or dizziness must undergo a complete evaluation to arrive at the correct diagnosis, which is then used to plan the treatment. The concepts of MCS can be used for diagnosis, where the *mechanics* phase consists of the evaluation of the reflexes, ocular and spinal, the *cybernetics* phase is the evaluation of the interaction of the subsystems, ocular and spinal, and, finally, the *synergetics* phase is the evaluation of the integration of functional networks.

From a practical point of view and because of the difficulty of distinguishing the individual contribution of each component (mechanics aspects) and each subsystem (cybernetics aspects) to the equilibrium performance, it is easier to divide the diagnostic approach to the patient into general and specific approaches. By general approach, we mean anamnesis and general clinical evaluation of the patient, and by specific approach we mean evaluation of the main functional levels of the equilibrium function: ocular, spinal and orientation.

3.1 General Approach

Anamnesis

In all medical fields a good evaluation of the case history is the key to correct diagnosis. The patient's complaints must be documented as completely as possible from the beginning of the disease. Sometimes the examiner uses technical terms to question the patient and this can lead to confusion and misinterpretations. The first diagnostic task is the differentiation between vertigo and dizziness or dysequilibrium, ruling out the many varieties of indistinct dizziness such as faintness. *Vertigo* is linked to a spinning sensation around the head and frequently is due to a vestibular disorder. It is the awareness of a

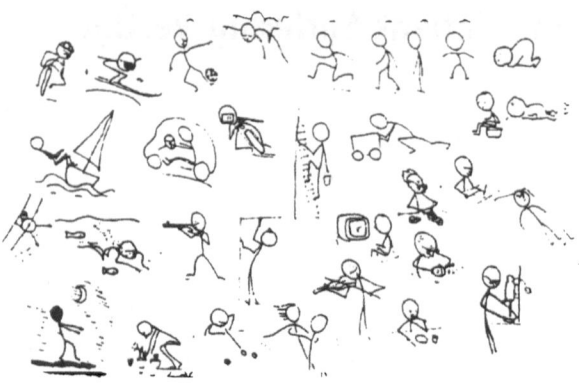

Fig. 3.1. Synoptic table of daily activities in which vertigo can occur, as proposed by Grateu (1992)

dysfunction in the balance mechanisms, that is, a dysfunction in the balance mechanisms becomes a conscious experience. The sensation is characterized by feelings of "spatial disorientation," of which the illusion of false movement is the most characteristic. "Rotatory sensation" is the most typical sensation, but it is not the sole feeling generated by balance dysfunction. The basic impression needs to be the sensation of loss of a stable subjective relationship with the environment. In this way less typical sensations must be included and are called "atypical" vertigo. On the other hand, syncopes, blackouts, drop attacks, odd sensations in the head, etc., need to be eliminated as primary "vertigo" sensations, but they can accompany true vertigo. *Dizziness* or a turning sensation inside the head may result from disturbances of integrating structures within the central nervous system. Atypical dizziness is usually confused with dysequilibrium. The term "dizziness" is used popularly and includes a multitude of symptoms related to the vestibular system or other aspects of the nervous system. Dizziness is applied to physical, emotional or intellectual disturbances, whose common denominator seems to be a loss of stability, a disruption of the pattern in which the individual is aware of his surroundings and their relation to him, whether these refer to his physical orientation in space, emotional equilibrium or intellectual clarity. It is important that the patient describes the symptoms with his or her own words in the simplest way. For this purpose Grateu proposed a simplified chart to investigate vertigo and dizziness during common or less common daily activities (Fig. 3.1). The examiner always needs to guide the patient in order to identify the main elements of the patient's history.

In equilibrium disturbances particular attention needs to be paid to the qualitative and quantitative aspects of the symptomatology.

Qualitative Aspects

The following aspects require investigation:
- Vertigo or dizziness. It is important to identify which symptom is prevalent, if both are present or if there is a particular and recurrent sequence between vertigo and dizziness. For example, after whiplash injury, dizziness appears when the patient removes the collar while performing normal activities, while vertigo appears during rotation or flexo-extension of the head.
- Onset of the symptoms.
- Direction of vertigo rotation or the side of prevalent unsteadiness.
- Remission with a particular position of the head/neck.
- Combination with spine pain and stiffness, with brachial paresthesias, with dysphagia or dysphasia, with neurovegetative symptoms such as nausea and vomiting, with cognitive symptoms such as amnesia and attentional disturbances, or with auditory symptoms such as hypoacusia and tinnitus.
- Loss of consciousness or combined with vertigo/dizziness.
- Headache and/or migraine immediately after a vertigo attack or in the following days/weeks/months.
- Incidence of symptoms during daily life activities. These qualitative aspects of the symptomatology can be quantified using activity daily life (ADL) questionnaires. As with functional scales, there is a tendency to use different standards, depending on the type of lesion one aims to study. However, the usefulness of a questionnaire and ADL estimations should not be underestimated. The clinician may well use this expertise to enhance the objective assessment of the patients. However, such estimations may be biased and they cannot easily be quantified or documented for studies or evaluation of the effect of treatment. To obtain better objective estimations, several functional scales have been developed, generally designed for the study of a certain group of patients, thereby lacking the quality of general applicability. Well-known scales are the Tinetti Subscale and the Balance Scale suggested by Berg.

Quantitative Aspects

- Temporal distance between any health disturbance and onset of symptomatology.
- Temporal onset of each symptom and reciprocal combination.
- Frequency of spontaneous attacks.
- Intensity, which can be quantified on a decimal scale.

- Duration: continuous, subcontinuous, transient, recurrent.
- Temporal correlation with hearing disturbances: no hearing disturbances, hearing symptoms before, during, and after vertigo attacks,
  etc.

In order to specify the relationship between symptoms and general
health status, concomitant diseases and disorders need to be investi-
gated:
- Previous trauma.
- Previous otoneurological visit/examinations either for symptoms or
  for a working capability evaluation.
- Previous auditory disorders.
- Heart, brain or vascular diseases.
- Hormonal disorders such as dysmenorrhea or dysthyroidism.
- Metabolic disorders such as diabetes.
- Use of alcohol, drugs and smoking.
- Exposure to solvents or other cerebrotoxic factors.
- Epilepsy.
- Previous treatment for scoliosis or correction of malocclusion, be-
  cause these problems can influence the possible treatments for
  compensation of the postural system.
- Kinetosis.

During anamnesis the manner in which the patient relates his own
history can suggest to the clinician other characteristics, such as anxiety, restlessness or depression. Sometimes specific psychometric
scales can be used, but they are generally not well accepted by the
subject. Computerized anamnestic systems, such as NODEC as described by Claussen, are very useful for standardizing the series of
questions, but they reduce the interpersonal interaction between clinician and patient. Generally speaking we can say that computerized
anamnestic systems are particularly indicated in medicolegal situations, while personal anamnesis is more useful in treatment planning.
The clinician needs to be able to identify psychological symptoms
due to stress and consequent symptoms. During anamnesis the examiner can, if necessary, simply evaluate attentional disturbances with
easy topical questions (today's date, etc.), cultural (name of the Pope,
etc.), memory (repeating a series of numbers, etc.) and logic reversal
ability tasks.

A useful questionnaire is the Dizziness Handicap Inventory (DHI)
proposed by Jacobs, Craig and Newman, of which a short form has
been recently developed by the present authors and Tesio. The DHI
investigates multiple aspects of daily activity and their correlation

Table 3.1. Dizziness Handicap Inventory developed by Jacobson, Craig and Newman (1990)

Instructions: the purpose of this scale is to identify difficulties that you may be experiencing *because of* your dizziness or unsteadiness. Please answer "yes," "no" or "sometimes" to each question. Answer each question as it pertains to your dizziness or unsteadiness problem only.

Does looking up increase your problem?
Because of your problem, do you feel frustrated?
Because of your problem, do you restrict your travel for business or recreation?
Does walking down the aisle of a supermarket increase your problem?
Because of your problem, do you have difficulty getting into or out of bed?
Does your problem significantly restrict your participation in social activities such as going out to dinner, going to movies, dancing or parties?
Because of your problem, do you have difficulties in reading?
Does performing more ambitious activities like sports, dancing, household chores such as sweeping or putting dishes away increase your problem?
Because of your problem, are you afraid to leave your home without having someone accompany you?
Because of your problem, have you been embarrassed in front of others?
Do quick movements of your head increase your problem?
Because of your problem, do you avoid heights?
Does turning over in bed increase your problem?
Because of your problem, is it difficult for you to do strenuous housework or yardwork?
Because of your problem are you afraid people may think you are intoxicated?
Because of your problem, is it difficult for you to go for a walk by yourself?
Does walking down a sidewalk increase your problem?
Because of your problem is it difficult to concentrate?
Because of your problem, is it difficult for you to walk around your house in the dark?
Because of your problem are you afraid to stay at home alone?
Because of your problem, do you feel handicapped?
Has your problem placed stress on your relationships with members of your family or friends?
Because of your problem, are you depressed?
Does your problem interfere with your job or household responsibilities?
Does bending over increase your problem?

with the evocation of equilibrium disturbances (Table 3.1). The short form is a simplified questionnaire which has been proved to be as reliable and accurate as the long form (Table 3.2). The questions are not restricted to the patient's problem (vertigo and dizziness) but they investigate the patient as an entire person. For example, it is possible that vertigo and dizziness do not cause difficulties in reading (answer "no" in the DHI) but the patient may suffer from vision impairment because of ophthalmological problems. In this case the cor-

Table 3.2. Dizziness Handicap Inventory, short form, modified by Tesio, Alpini, Cesarani and Perucca (1998)

Instructions: the purpose of this scale is to identify difficulties that you may be experiencing that can cause your dizziness or unsteadiness. Please answer "yes" or "no" to each question *even if* disturbances are caused by problems different from vertigo, dizziness and unsteadiness.
Does looking up increase your symptoms?
Do you restrict your travel for business or recreation?
Do you have difficulty getting into or out of bed?
Do you have difficulties in reading?
Do quick movements of your head increase your problem?
Do you avoid heights?
Does turning over in bed increase your problem?
Is it difficult for you to go for a walk by yourself?
Does walking down a sidewalk increase your problem?
Is it difficult for you to walk around your house in the dark?
Are you afraid to stay at home alone?
Are you depressed?
Does bending over increase your problem?

rect answer in the DHI will be "yes" because reading is difficult and the impaired vision, for any reason, may impair balance.

General Clinical Examination

Cranial Nerves

Generally, the olfactory nerve is not investigated routinely because it requires specialized equipment (olfactometry). The opticus nerve can be clinically investigated, with evaluation of the fundus oculi by means of an ophthalmoscope. Extrinsic and intrinsic ocular motility always needs to be investigated. During oculomotricity, smooth pursuit and saccadic eye movements need to be investigated using a pen or the examiner's finger as the target. Also the sensitivity of the face (trigeminus) and the corneal reflexes needs to be evaluated. Regarding the facial nerve, facial aspects are sometimes evident and dysesthesias of the auditory external meatus need to be looked for. The Shirmer test can be used to complete the facial examination. Auditory function is best investigated with the different audiometric tests, leaving the diapason tests to the history. Only the Weber test can be sometimes useful during the clinical investigation. Inspection of the mouth and the larynx enables a complete evaluation of the IX, X and XII nerves to be made, which can be completed with stimulation of the external auditory meatus and posterior pharyngeal wall to induce pharyngeal reflexes. The XI nerve is usually evaluated during the posture examination, with palpation of the sternocleidomastoidus and trapezius muscles.

Posture Evaluation

Several approaches may be used to estimate human postural control and they may be considered complementary. Clinical investigation can yield valuable information. The direct observation of patient behavior, even during anamnesis, may contribute information which may otherwise be overlooked. Several generally well known examination procedures may be applied to help the examiner evaluate the investigated subject. The use of standardized protocols also gives the examiner more experience in interpreting the outcome of the procedures. The active and passive movements of the head with respect to the neck, the trunk and the pelvis must be estimated. Pain and movement limitations have to be noted and in a certain way quantified. Palpations of paravertebral extensory muscles, with special regard to those of the neck and the back, need to be performed in order to appreciate hypo- or hypertonus of the muscles. A simple muscular force test for the arm and leg extensory muscles is useful. With the patient in the supine position, a Babinsky test is simple and useful to perform. General muscular tonus can be simply evaluated by asking to the patient to form a ring with his or her thumb and index finger and the examiner trying to open this ring.

Tendon reflexes may be simply investigated. Trigger and tender points need to be routinely searched for along all the paravertebral muscles and the temporomandibular joint needs to be inspected in static and dynamic (opening, protrusion, laterotrusion, etc.) positions of the jaw.

During postural evaluation some sensorial evaluation can be simultaneously performed especially if paresthesias are complained of.

3.2 Specific Approach: Ocular Function

Eye Movements

Eye movements can easily be evaluated in a clinical manner using the appropriate instrumentation. In clinical practice the investigator stands in front of the patient. First the examiner suddenly lifts the right thumb in front of the patient (about 50 cm from the patient's eyes) asking him to fixate it without moving his head, then he lifts the left thumb. The examiner continues lifting alternately the right and left thumbs and the patient continues fixating them, producing saccadic eye movements. The most important features that can be noted are the latency of the eye movements and their conjugation. Also dysmetrias can be revealed because sometimes patients are not able to fixate the thumb with only one saccade, but they require adjustment of the eye movements. The examiner then asks the patient to fixate his right thumb placed at 50 cm from the patient's eyes, during a slow continuous to-and-fro movement. In this case a smooth pursuit can be elicited. The most important feature that can be noted is the regularity of the movement, which must be continuous and harmonic.

For instrumental evaluation, the most common technique is electro-oculography (EOG), which is based on the so-called corneoretinal potential: the corneoretinal axis is a bipolar axis in which the positive pole is the cornea and the negative one is the retina. This axis is the same as the visual axis. The corneoretinal potential is about 1 mV. If two electrodes are placed on the skin corresponding to the inner and outer canthi, it is possible to record the movements of the eyes as a variation of the position of the corneoretinal axis. A computer analyzes and elaborates the data in order to present graphic traces and calculations regarding the eye movements.

Other techniques do exist such as recording by means of magnetic search coils and infrared recording. These techniques are usually employed in basic research and are very rarely used in the clinical field. The most modern technique for recording eye movements is video-oculography (VOG). A video camera directly records the movements of the eyes and a computer analyzes the data obtained in this way. Compared with EOG, VOG is more accurate during the evaluation of torsional eye movements. Table 3.3 presents a summary of the main advantages and disadvantages of the systems used for recording eye movements and nystagmus. For the investigation of a patient with a balance disorder in whom an investigation of vestibular responses is required, the technique generally recommended is EOG as it allows recordings over a wide range of amplitudes, it is the cheapest system and it does not require a great deal of technical and scientific support. It is mainly used for investigation of horizontal eye movements and therefore for assessment of horizontal semicircular canal function. It can produce some reasonable recordings in the vertical plane but it is totally insensitive to torsional movements.

Table 3.3. Advantages and disadvantages of different eye movement recordings

	Electro-oculography (EOG/ENG)	Infrared oculography	Scleral search coil
Signal source	Corneoretinal potential	Limbus infrared light refraction	Contact lens-mounted search coil
Advantages	Noninvasive; simple and inexpensive; prolonged recordings; good linearity	Noninvasive	Excellent resolution
Disadvantages	Low-resolution noise; drift	Poor linearity; moderately expensive	Invasive torsional recordings; expensive

Eye movements are elicited by visual targets during both EOG and VOG. Targets can be presented either on a light-emitting diode (LED) bar or projected on a screen. Saccades are elicited by sudden displacement of a target, while smooth pursuit is elicited by a continuous smooth displacement of the target.

For saccades the following parameters are investigated:
- Latency: the difference between the displacement of the target and the displacement of the eye
- Accuracy: how the ocular movement is accurate in positioning the eye exactly on the target
- Velocity: proportional to the width of the target displacement.

The results are usually compared with normal values evaluated in a control population.

In Fig. 3.2 a normal horizontal saccadic pattern is shown, while in Fig. 3.3 a hypermetric saccadic pattern caused by a lesion of the cerebellum is seen.

For smooth pursuit the following parameters are generally investigated:
- Maximum velocity: the most common pattern is a sinusoidal displacement of the target. Thus it is possible to calculate both a maximum and mean velocity.
- Gain: this is the ratio between mean velocity of the target and the ocular movement. It indicates the effectiveness of the ocular motor performance.
- Offset: this indicates the symmetry of the movement. In some cases smooth pursuit can be conserved in one direction and altered in the other.

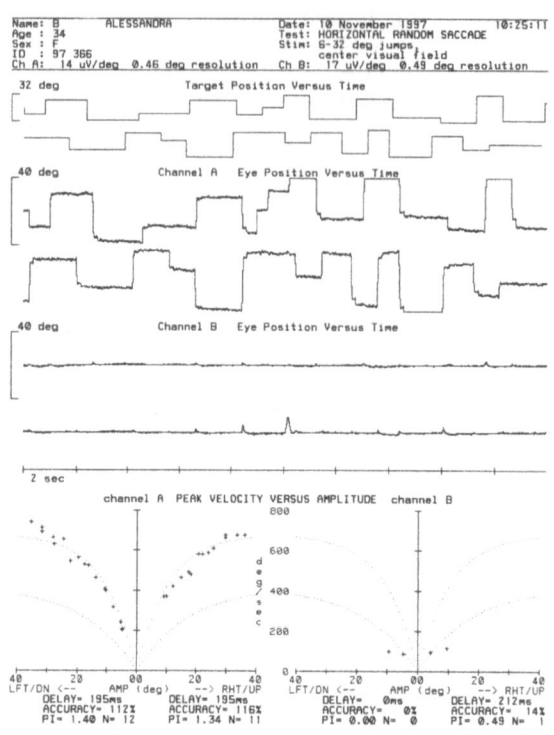

Fig. 3.2. Normal horizontal saccades. The first trace refers to the target, the second to horizontal bitemporal recording, the third to monocular vertical recording

- Distortion: this indicates if the movement is a smooth movement or if the patients need interposed corrective saccades to reach and maintain the target position.
- Phase: this indicates how many of the eye movements are regular and the ocular delay in respect of the target.

In Fig. 3.4 a normal horizontal smooth pursuit pattern is shown. Figure 3.5 shows a normal vertical smooth pursuit pattern.

Vestibulo-ocular Reflex

Clinically, information on the vestibulo-ocular reflex (VOR) can be obtained by turning the patient's head while observing the optic disk during funduscopy. The patient must be instructed to maintain fixation on an object across the room. Normally, the disk remains steady in space but if, for example, the right labyrinth is hypoactive, the disk will seem to jerk during turning of the head to the right. When the vestibular loss is profound, this jerky eye movement in response

Fig. 3.3. Hypermetric saccades. The recording shows that accuracy is higher than in the normal pattern

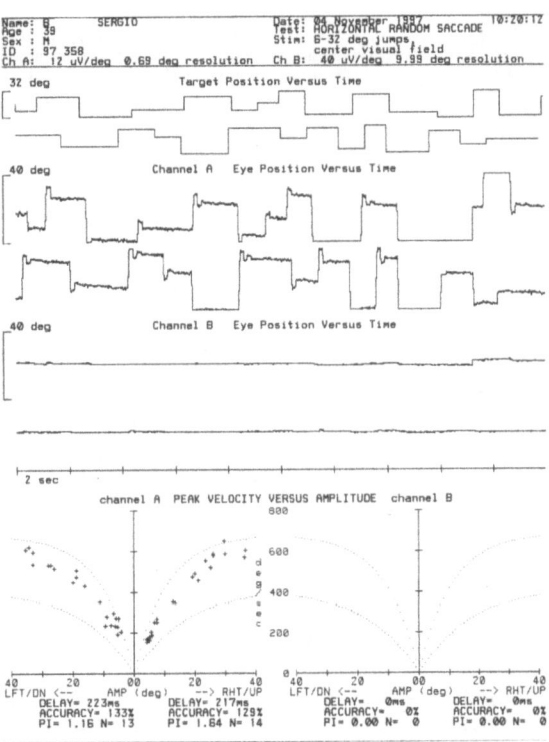

to turns of the head can be seen by the naked eye. In this case it is best to instruct the patient to fixate on the examiner's nose (the so-called Halmagyi sign).

Assessment of the otolith function clinically is even less easily done. Counter rolling of the eyes can be seen when the head is rotated to ear down on to the shoulder; the eyes slowly deviate in the opposite direction and then there is a rotatory quick phase causing torsional nystagmus. This response is, however, mainly dependent on the vertical semicircular canals rather than the otoliths. Skew deviation of the eyes (vertical divergence of the eyes) without nystagmus is thought to reflect tonic otolith pathway imbalance. It can be seen with utricular nerve lesion or with lesions of the mesencephalon, especially those involving the interstitial nucleus of Cajal and medulla; this type of tonic rotation can be suspected from a head tilt or the eye-covering test or can be seen from tilting of the optic disk.

One of the cardinal signs of abnormal vestibular function is *nystagmus* (Ny), which is a biphasic involuntary movement of both eyes

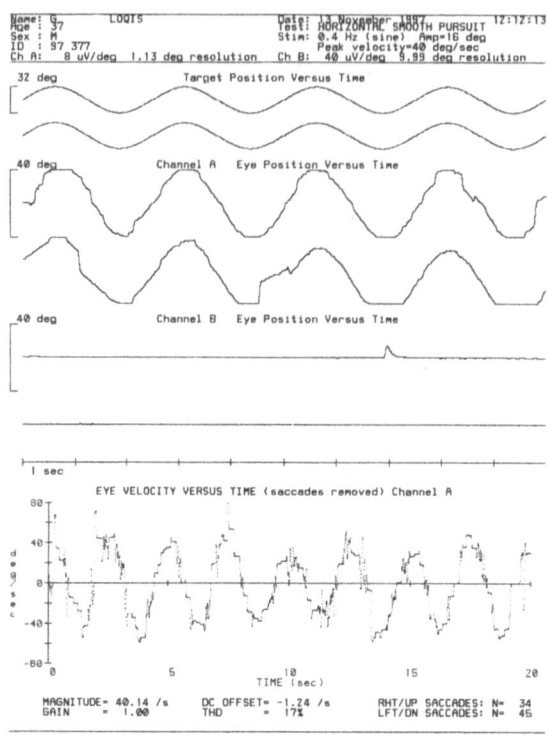

Fig. 3.4. Normal horizontal smooth pursuit

(generally) and consists of a slow displacement of the eyes in one direction (slow phase of nystagmus) followed by a rapid return of the eyes in the primary position of the gaze. EOG and VOG are the specific instrumental techniques used to record and analyze nystagmus (electronystagmography and video-nystagmography).

Nystagmus is classified according to the maneuvers that are able to elicit it:

1. Spontaneous nystagmus is present without any provocative maneuver.
2. Vestibular nystagmus is caused by an imbalance between the paired vestibular structures. The nystagmus is called first degree if present only when the gaze is directed towards the fast phase, second degree if present in the primary position, or third degree if present when the eyes are deviated in the direction of the slow phase. Removal of fixation typically enhances the nystagmus if the lesion is peripheral and the eyes drift markedly towards the deranged side (fast phase towards the healthy side). This can be seen clinically with Frenzel's glasses, which have high-diopter convergence lenses

Fig. 3.5. Normal vertical smooth pursuit

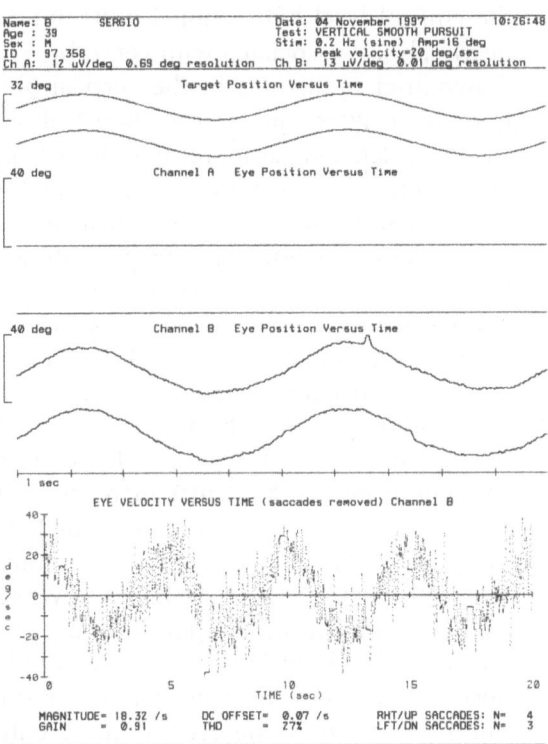

that allow a magnified view of the eyes of the patient, without the patient being able to fixate due to the blur produced by the lenses.

The typical pattern of recorded nystagmus (by ENG or VNG) is sawtoothed with a linear (constant) velocity, slow phase. With gaze paretic nystagmus the slow phase has a roughly exponential decline interrupted by repeated fast phases. This form of nystagmus is due to failure of integration of the burst of activity arising from the saccadic generators in the paramedian pontine reticular formation (PPRF). This results in insufficient tonic holding activity to maintain the eyes in the eccentric position against the orbital elastic forces, tending to return the eye to the orbital mid-position. Failure of integration most commonly occurs in lesions of the brainstem and cerebellum but can also be seen if there is a failure of faithful transmission of activity through the final common pathway of the extraocular muscles or if the muscles themselves are unable to contract effectively. This form of nystagmus occurs in a wide variety of CNS conditions, many of which are associated with imbalance. At the clinical level bidirectional nystagmus in the horizontal plane is nearly always associated with central dysfunction.

Acquired nystagmus in the vertical plane occurs less often than horizontal nystagmus and is almost always an indication of a central disorder. Furthermore, it is invariably accompanied by imbalance. Vertical upbeat nystagmus, especially if present in the primary position, indicates a lesion in the floor of the IVth ventricle or ventral to the aqueduct, or possibly within the superior cerebellar vermis; it is often seen in patients with bilateral internuclear ophthalmoplegia. Downbeat nystagmus is seen with lesions at the foramen magnum, for example, Arnold-Chiari malformation, or cerebellar atrophy. Characteristically vertical nystagmus is altered by position and downbeat nystagmus is increased in amplitude if the eyes are deviated 30° to the left or right of the midline.

2. Nystagmus evoked by ocular maneuvers: there are two kinds of this nystagmus. The most common is elicited by the eccentric position of the eyes that the patient has to maintain for at least 20 s. It is also called gaze-evoked nystagmus. When bilateral, it is usually a sign of central disorders due to a deficit of the central gaze neural integrator localized in the medial vestibular nucleus and in the prepositus hypoglossi nucleus. The other type is rebound nystagmus. The patient moves the eyes in an eccentric position. A nystagmus is observed. Then the patient returns his or her eyes to the primary position and a nystagmus towards the opposite side is observed. When bilateral, it is due to an archicerebellar dysfunction.

3. Positional nystagmus: nystagmus may be readily induced, or, if already present, modified by changes in position of the head. The conventional method is the Hallpike maneuver. In this, the patient sits on a couch and the examiner firmly grasps the head, which is turned 60° towards one shoulder. The patient is instructed to keep the eyes open and to fixate the examiner's forehead. The patient's head is rapidly lowered to below the level of the couch and the eyes observed for any nystagmus. After an interval of 30 s, if nystagmus is not found, or after the nystagmus ceases, the patient is returned to the sitting position. Again, any nystagmus is normally noted. The test is repeated if nystagmus is found to see if there is any adaptation. After this, the test is performed with the opposite ear dependent. The variables noted are latency to onset of nystagmus, its duration and adaptation, its direction, and, finally, associated symptoms. If any nystagmus is found after the Hallpike maneuver, nystagmus needs to be investigated for with the patient in the supine position, in the head-hanging position (Rose's maneu-

ver) and with brisk turning of the head to one side while the patient is in the supine position (MacClure's maneuver). Typical benign positional nystagmus indicates a peripheral dysfunction, it presents a latency, it is generally horizontal-rotatory, and it is usually geotropic, fatigable and adaptable. Although it is generally unilateral, occasionally what seems to be bilateral benign positional nystagmus occurs.

Typical central positional nystagmus occurs in a wide variety of lesions, especially those involving vestibulocerebellum. Of note is the fact that spontaneous vertical nystagmus, either upwards or downwards, can often be modified by positional testing using the conventional Hallpike maneuver or by placing the subject supine or prone. If the nystagmus is increased with the patient in the prone position it is usually decreased with the patient lying supine. Nystagmus induced by canal stimulation can also be profoundly modified by alteration of the position of the head, due to otolith/semicircular canal interaction.

4. Nystagmus induced by stimulation of the semicircular canals: Two methods are available to stimulate the semicircular canals: caloric testing and rotational stimuli. Caloric nystagmus depends primarily on the convection set-up in the relevant canal by thermal stimulation. Irrigation of the external meatus sets up a convection current, which flows upwards if hot water is used and stimulates the hair cells; conversely the cold stimulus causes movement of the endolymph away from the ampulla and reduces the firing rate of the cells. In Fig. 3.6 a typical caloric cold response is shown. Thermal stimulation of hair cells without any convection would also cause similar effects on the hair cell firing rate, but in fact this probably only accounts for a small proportion of the alteration although it accounts for all of it in conditions of zero gravity such as space travel. The nystagmic response is used to assess the effect of canal irrigation. Nystagmus is induced to the side opposite the irrigated ear in the case of cold irrigation and vice versa for warm irrigation.

The main parameters are: (a) duration of the nystagmus response, (b) mean slow-phase velocity or frequency of nystagmus beats during the period of maximum response (culmination), and (c) symmetry of the response. In this case Jongkees elaborated two formula to calculate, on the basis of two cold and two hot irrigations, if a directional preponderance or a canal paresis exists. In fact three types of abnormalities are seen with horizontal canal irrigation. Firstly, there may be an underfunctioning of one canal, con-

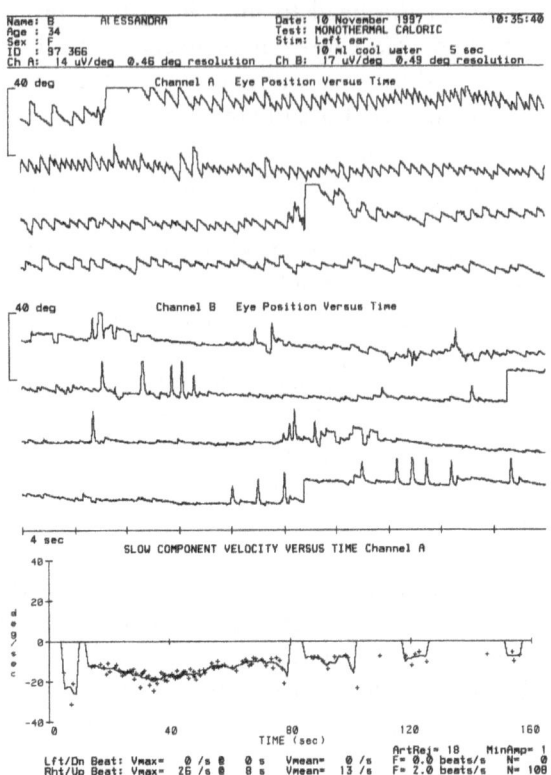

Fig. 3.6. Normal caloric response to left cold stimulation

ventionally called "canal paresis." This typically occurs in peripheral lesions and a total failure of function of one horizontal canal is nearly always due to end organ or VIIIth nerve damage. Secondly, there may be a bias of nystagmus such that the frequency or the mean slow phase velocity in one direction, for example the left (with right cold and left hot irrigation), is greater than that to the opposite side. This is known as directional preponderance and can be seen in peripheral disorders as well as with lesions at any level of the nervous system. It does, however, show thereby a vestibular bias in one direction and if there is a canal paresis as well it indicates that this is not fully compensated. Finally, there may be hypofunction of both horizontal canals, for example, after aminoglycoside antibiotic treatment.

Caloric testing can also be used to assess the function of the vertical canals but in this case only pairs of canals, either anterior or posterior, are studied. These canals are set deeper in the petrous temporal bone than the horizontal canals and therefore a longer duration and more intense thermal stimuli are required. Both ears are irrigated simultaneously with either cold or hot water for 60 s with the head in the usual position for caloric testing. The cold stimulus causes slow downward deviation of the eyes with upbeat nystagmus and the hot stimulus the reverse.

During caloric testing it is possible to assess visual suppression of nystagmus (Visual Suppression Test, VST) without contamination from other reflex eye movements. A practicable method is to perform each irrigation in the dark or under Frenzel's glasses and to instruct the patient to fixate a small target (generally a small light) immediately after the period of culmination. Comparing the mean slow-phase velocities during culmination and during fixation it is possible to calculate an index of visual suppression (Index of Ocular Fixation). In cases of central lesions, especially those involving cerebellar connections, visual suppression is reduced or absent so that there is pronounced nystagmus with fixation. This further important finding that can be made on the VOR may be performed also in a clinical setting. The VST is easily tested by getting the subject to fixate a long spatula gripped in the teeth while oscillating the head in the horizontal or vertical plane, or more simply by fixating the thumbs with arms outstretched while rotating at the wrist or on a wheelchair. No nystagmus is seen in normal subjects until the frequency of oscillation approaches 1 Hz or the peak velocity is greater than $60°/s$.

It is possible to obtain reliable and quantitative information on vestibular function using a motorized chair. Two variables are used to define *rotational stimuli*: the waveform of the stimulus, whether sinusoidal, trapezoidal, or square wave (impulsive), and the peak velocity reached during rotation. Trapezoidal stimulation induces a constant liminal acceleration of the chair until a constant velocity is reached. The constant velocity rotation is maintained until the nystagmic response disappears and the patient is stopped with a sudden deceleration. After the induced nystagmus ceases, the patient is rotated in the opposite direction so that two sets of right-beating responses (right start and stop from the left) and two left-beating (left start and stop from the right) are collected. Responses can be expressed in terms of duration, peak slow-phase velocity achieved, or time constant of decay of initial peak velocity, that is, time to decay to about one-third of the induced velocity, or by a combination of these. If the stimulus is sinusoidal (constant and continuous acceleration and deceleration), it is important that a

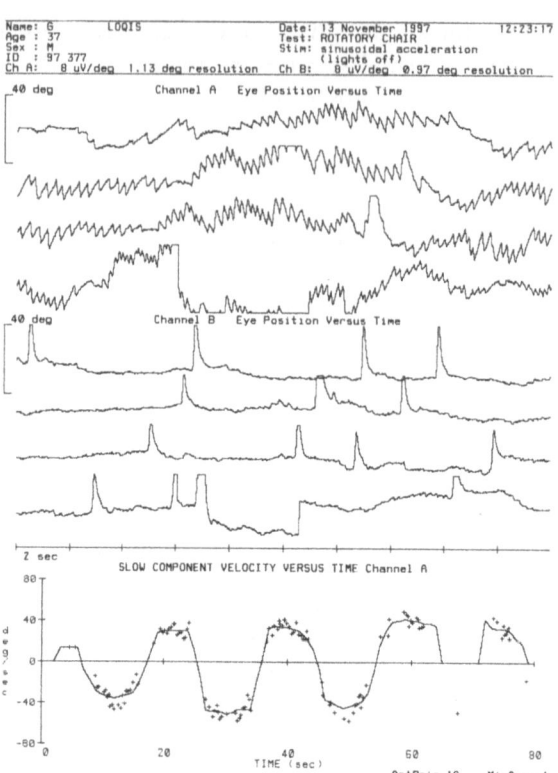

Fig. 3.7. Normal response to sinusoidal stimulation

range, rather than a single, frequency is tested to achieve a thorough investigation of the vestibular ocular system. In Fig. 3.7 a typical normal sinusoidal response is shown, while Fig. 3.8 shows a disconjugate response to sinusoidal stimulation that shows differences in maximum and mean slow-phase velocity in rightward movements of the right eye and leftward eye movements of the left eye.

A useful addition to the sinusoidal rotational test is to determine suppression of the VOR during rotation and contemporary fixation of a target attached to the chair (usually a small light); thus the patient fixates an object that moves with him during the oscillations. Another useful test is stimulation of the visuo-VOR (VVOR), which is rotation with eyes open to the light. The gain of VOR is generally lower than 1 unit (0.6–0.8), while during rotation in the light visual pathways provide information necessary to allow a complete recov-

Fig. 3.8. In these recordings the upper traces refer to the right eye while the lower traces refer to the left eye. The pattern is that of internuclear ophthalmoplegia with slowing of the adducting eye (left in rightward movements and vice versa)

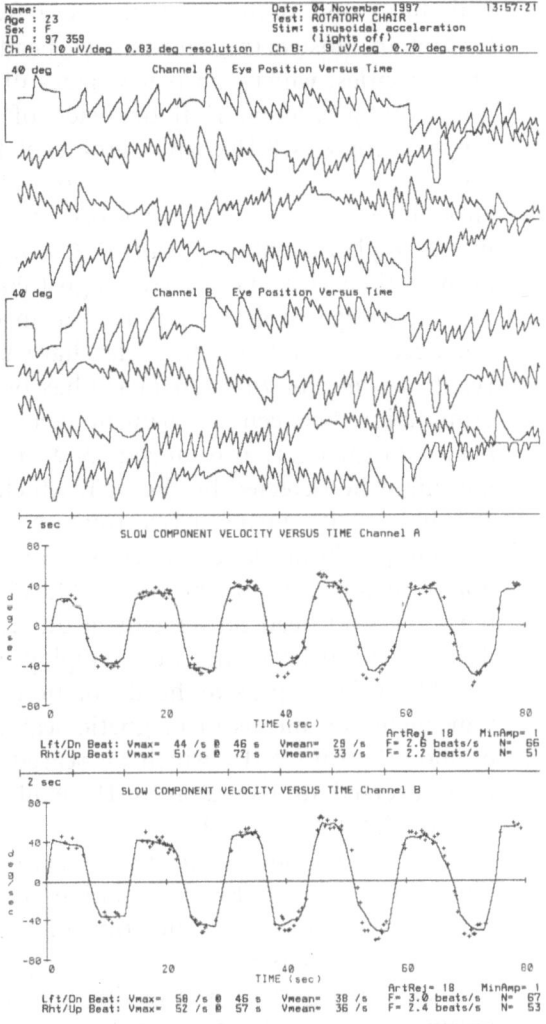

ery of gain velocity up to 1. Comparing slow phase velocity (SPV) during rotation in the dark (VOR) and light (VVOR), the clinician is able to gather important information regarding the efficiency of the whole oculomotor subsystem.

Most clinical rotatory tests employed are conducted at oscillation frequencies up to 0.5 Hz. The 0.5-Hz limit is imposed by the torque limit of the motor driving the chair and problems concerned with head and body fixation. These frequencies are below those present in most active and passive head movements during everyday activities, which can reach values of at least 6 Hz. During running, the predominant frequencies of head rotations may even range as high as 8 Hz, with significant harmonics up to 15 Hz. In this frequency range, the visual control system has a large influence. Therefore the search has been for tests to measure the VOR in the higher frequency range. A fairly recent development has been both active and passive high-frequency head rotation tests. The advantage of these tests is that an expensive rotatory chair is not necessary and results so far have been promising. The *active vestibular autorotation test (VAT)* has been postulated to allow discrimination between an acoustic neuroma and Meniere's disease from a normal ear; also the side and the size of the acoustic neuroma might be detected by the VAT, which consists of a recording of eye movements during active rotation of the head at different frequencies, in both planes. A rate sensor on a headband or on a bite board records movements of the head. Dedicated software compares eye and head movements at different frequencies. A specially designed headshaker has been employed by Collewijn et al. in order to evaluate passive head rotation, measuring eye and head movements by means of magnetic search coils. They report a gain of about 1 from 2 Hz, which decreased at 8 Hz but then the VOR gain reversed to 1.1–1.3 at 20 Hz while phase lag increased from zero to about $45°$ at 20 Hz.

5. Cervical nystagmus is due to the activation of the cervico-ocular reflex. It is elicited by the rotation of the subject with the head still. This provokes a stimulation of the neck muscles (stretching reflex), a stimulation of the vestibular nuclei and the elicitation of a nystagmus directed towards the opposite side of body rotation. In normal subjects nystagmus does not usually appear; thus the gain of the COR has been calculated to be very low (about 0.1). In patients cervical nystagmus can be more easily observed especially when the labyrinth is hypofunctional.

6. Head-shaking nystagmus: In some patients vigorous head shaking may generate a nystagmus that is not clinically apparent. The head-shaking test (HST) (20–30 full cycles at around 2 Hz followed by observation with Frenzel's glasses) is claimed to be a useful addition to the clinical vestibular examination.

7. Optokinetic nystagmus (OKN) (Fig. 3.9) is a nystagmus elicited by rotation of the environment with respect to the patient. It is a compensatory movement of the eyes to pursue a target displacement of

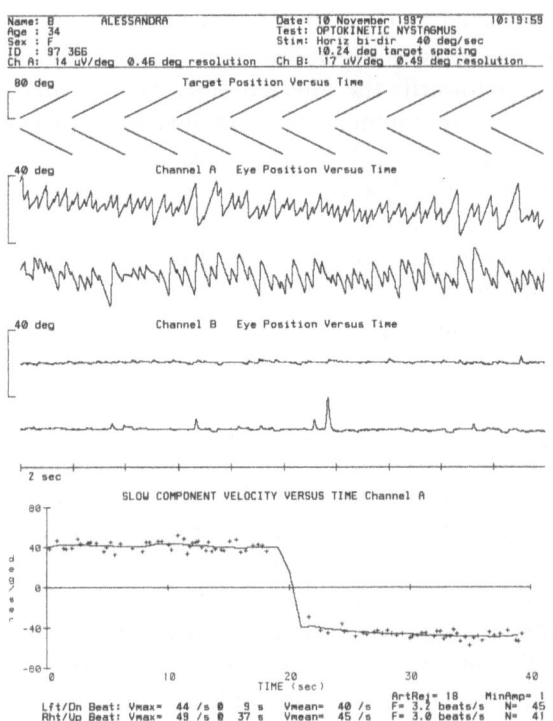

Fig. 3.9. Normal bitemporal recording of optokinetic nystagmus

greater width than the visual field. It can be assessed at the bedside with a small striped drum rotated in front of the patient. This is basically a pursuit task and not surprisingly correlates well with other pursuit measures. It is possible to measure OKN with a small drum, or with a large visual field rotating about the patient using various special techniques such as electronystagmography (ENG). A common abnormality is directional preponderance – that is, a greater response in one direction. Typically a right directional preponderance correlates with abnormal pursuit to the right (for example, a right cerebellar or parietal lesion results in greater OKN towards the right). In a normal subject the eyes deviate in the direction of the fast phase of OKN but in certain disorders of the basal ganglia the converse happens, that is, deviation is in the direction of the slow phase. Regarding unilateral vestibular hypofunction, a directional preponderance of OKN is usually observed. In the early phases of the disease, OKN is preponderant toward the side of spontaneous nystagmus. During compensation three situations may occur: no directional preponderance, directional preponderance towards the affected side, or directional preponderance towards the healthy side. A good compensation process requires a directional preponderance towards the affected side. This means that nystagmogenic processes are compensated and this kind of asymmetry is the same as the so-called recovery nystagmus, that is a spontaneous nystagmus directed towards the hypofunctional labyrinth. Vertical OKN is usually asymmetrical: upward OKN is generally wider and faster than downward OKN and this is due to the influence of otolithic inputs to the vestibular nuclei that interferes with the production of nystagmus.

Otolith Function

Some patients attending balance disorder clinics report symptoms of unsteadiness which suggest involvement of the otolith rather than semicircular canal function. This may include a sense of bobbing up and down, being carried upwards and downwards in a lift, or lateral and sagittal pulsions. Certain disorders of head and eye coordination – for instance, the ocular tilt reaction combining head tilt and ocular skew deviation – are thought to be due to interruption of central graviceptive otolith pathways. Despite all the clinical evidence, reliable and simple tests for otolith function in human are lacking. This is due to the difficulties in delivering the appropriate stimuli (whole body tilt or linear acceleration) which require large motion devices and the simultaneous recording of a meaningful response (ocular torsion), which requires eye coils or video-oculography. The only technique which does not require extraordinary equipment to investigate otolith function is eccentric rotation of the subject. In this procedure the subject's head is placed eccentrically in front of the axis of rotation of a conventional rotating chair while horizontal eye movements are recorded with standard techniques. The rationale is that in this position the head experiences not only angular acceleration but also a tangential component along the interaural axis, which gives rise to stimulation of the utricular macula. The enhanced VOR elicited in this position has been proved in experimental animals to be due to otolith stimulation. Although clinical abnormalities can be detected, full evaluation in the clinical setting has not been undertaken.

3.3 Specific Approach: Spinal Function

Stance

Most common human activities require the ability to stabilize the human body in upright stance, to counteract perturbations and to allow voluntary movements, according to gravitational forces. The standing human is an unstable physical structure. To counteract the effects of gravity and comply with the requirements to stabilize the body during voluntary movements, there is a continuous modulation of motor activity, especially in the so-called antigravity muscles, based on the also continuously changing afferent sensory information. The postural control of the standing human can therefore be considered in part to be a dynamic feedback control. Furthermore, based on experience and visual information, the standing human may foresee perturbations or changing requirements in advance, thus adding a substantial degree of anticipatory or feed-forward control. To evaluate the significance on postural control of observations or test results, it is necessary to bear in mind the physiological background and ability to maintain an upright stance. Regarding the clinical evaluation of stance, the classical Romberg test is easily applied even in the office and may yield some information. A patient unable to perform a Romberg test will probably have major difficulties in everyday life. During this test particular attention needs to be paid to the direction of the slow-falling rather than the fast compensation. The Romberg test with the feet in the tandem position seems less appropriate as it requires a better than ordinary postural control and will yield a high degree of false-positive results. A Romberg test with the neck extended, however, may contribute further information. In this position the lateral semicircular canal is brought into line with the gravity vector. A patient with a vestibular lesion causing ataxia and nystagmus falls in the direction of the slow phase of nystagmus, while a patient with a cerebellar disorder may fall toward the fast phase or the slow phase depending on the site of the lesion. According to Magnusson (1994), a combination of the clinical headshake test and the Romberg test may be performed. Nystagmus induced by a headshake test cannot differentiate between a CNS lesion or a peripheral vestibular lesion. One may, however, increase the sensitivity in tests of stance by combining the headshake test with a Romberg or a stepping test. The patient does headshakes for 10 s, standing with his back against a wall, then rapidly taking four steps forwards. If there is an evident deviation or the patient falls toward the side of the fast phase of nystagmus in-

Force-plate Design   Fig. 3.10. The principles of stabilometry

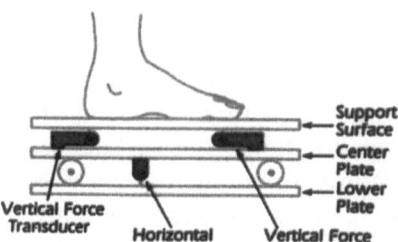

duced by a previous headshake test, this may be taken as suggesting a posterior fossa lesion. Patients with compensated peripheral vestibular lesions seem to deviate only slightly.

Measurement of body movements to quantitatively and objectively evaluate postural control and responses led to the development of different sets of *posturography*. The basic concept of this depends on the measurement of the forces actuated by the feet against the ground, measured with a forceplate. The forceplate consists of force tranducers placed to pick up the distribution of forces which are vertical or horizontal to the ground (Fig. 3.10). The simultaneous recordings from several transducers allows calculation of the moment produced by the standing human in different directions and shear (or transitional) forces to normalize the effects of weight of different subjects. The data may then be used to calculate the projection of forces against the ground. It is of the utmost importance to the understanding of posturography to realize that the recorded projection of all the forces against the ground is not the same as a projection of the subject center of mass (or gravity) but just the center of forces. The trace that is recorded is thus not equivalent to movements, especially fast ones, but rather to the stabilizing forces.

Different variables may be derived from the force measurements. The sway amplitude, sway variance, of sway in either the anteroposterior or lateral planes or sway path, sway velocity and sway area describing two-dimensional movements are commonly used variables to evaluate postural competence. In Fig. 3.11, a normalized test results diagram performed by Balance Master (Neurocom, Clackamas, Oregon, USA) is shown. The test has been evaluated under three conditions, eyes open, eyes closed and with visual feedback. The parameters calculated were sway and average position with reference to an ideal position of the CoG on the basis of the age and height of the patient. The results are shown as percentiles of normal values.

Fig. 3.11. An example of stabilometric normalized results with regard to sway and average position. (Balance Master, reproduced with courtesy of NeuroCom International, Inc., Clackamas, Oregon, USA)

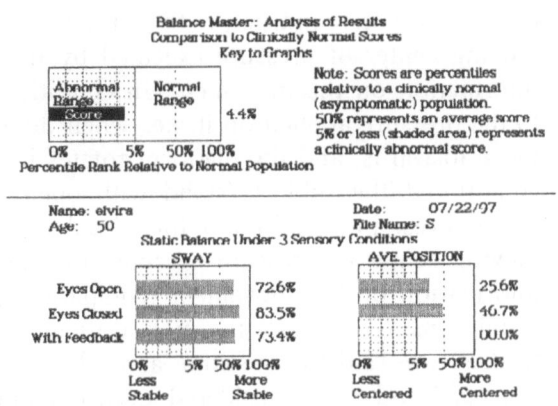

Although measurements of quiet stance may contribute to separation of groups of subjects with different lesions, the normal variations are so wide that classification of individual responses, and hence clinical usefulness, becomes ambiguous. To master such shortcomings, different techniques to increase the demands on postural control are applied. The idea is that if there is a deficit in the postural control system that is not evident because of the redundancy and adaptability of the systems, the deficit will become evident if further sensory information is lost or distorted. The classical Romberg test uses evasion of visual clues to load the postural system. Likewise, posturography can be performed and results compared with open and closed eyes. This is a standard procedure used in most test set-ups. If the increase in sway compared to normals is greater with open eyes than with closed eyes, this might be taken as suggesting less effective use of visual clues and may be, but not unequivocally, interpreted as a sign of decreased CNS function (so-called postural blindness). A foam rubber pad can be positioned between the feet of the subject and the forceplate to reduce mechanoreceptor sensation from the soles of the feet and increase the difficulty of stabilizing the body. The patient can be asked to place his head in different positions to increase the difficulty of vestibular cervical interaction.

The sensory integration tests of the *Equitest* (Neurocom, Clackamas, Oregon, USA) equipment, which is probably the most widespread commercially available system, utilize six sets of disturbed sensory information to estimate a sensory integration set. In conditions 1, 2 and 3 the subjects stand on a stable platform and the anteroposterior sway is estimated as a percentage of maximal sway. In condition 1 the subjects stand with open eyes; in condition 2 with closed eyes; in condition 3 the visual surroundings move with the moving center of pressure executed by the feet to distort the visual information on the movement. In conditions 4–6 the platform reacts to the pressure applied on it, i.e., when the forces actuated by the feet move forwards, and the platform rotates in a toes-down direction. In condition 4 the subjects stand with open eyes; in condition 5 with closed eyes; in condition 6 the visual surroundings move with the moving center of pressure executed by the feet to distort the visual information on the movement (compare with conditions 1–3 above). Conditions 5 and 6 are the most difficult to endure and poor results in these are said to constitute a vestibular pattern. Deficits in conditions 3, 5 and 6 are considered a sensory integration deficit.

To further load human postural control with the purpose of revealing deficits, the standing subject may be exposed to different perturbations and the responses to recover quiet stance are evaluated. In the T-Post system from Toennies (Wurzburg), the subjects stand, leaning somewhat backwards; the platform then tilts and induces a further backwards movement of the body. The subjects have to move forward to avoid falling; latencies and amplitudes of this movement can be combined with EMG recordings to estimate response latencies. The method can detect movement and probe synergistic muscle activity if combined with EMG. In the motor coordination test of the Equitest, the platform is either tilted or translated with different velocities and the postural reactions of the subject are measured. Vibration toward the antigravity muscles induces a sensation of movement and involuntary body movements. This has been used to perturb the standing human for diagnostic purposes, calculating vibration-induced body sway (VBS). Patients with posterior fossa lesions are reported to have larger responses when vibrated toward neck muscles than calf muscles, compared to subjects with vestibular lesions. Vibration toward the calf muscles according to a pseudorandom binary stimulus (PRBS) induces an on- and off-going perturbation which can be used to estimate an input-output relation and model postural control, which allows estimation of so-called characteristic parameters of postural control. Comparing these parameters, one can obtain an estimation of the postural control of the subject. Recently, it has been suggested that the use of these parameters can distinguish, for example, between an acoustic neurinoma and an acute vestibular lesion and can also distinguish subjects with cervical disorders. Patients who recover from hemispheric stroke demonstrate remaining differences in postural control when evaluated with these parameters. A vestibular spinal perturbation may evoke both lateral and anteroposterior body sway by galvanic stimulation of the vestibular nerves. Evaluation of these responses may give further information on posterior fossa lesions, but so far clinical studies are lacking. Visual stimulation inducing a sensation of small-amplitude translatory movements of the surroundings may induce perturbations in the anteroposterior plane, which, not surprisingly, differs in subjects with cerebellar lesions. The effect of visual stimulation, however, may be dependent on attention and state of mind and different patterns of response may be assumed in normal subjects. So far visually induced perturbations, with the exception of the so-called stabilized visual frame in Equitest measurements, have not been used in clinical routine.

Gait

Gait is certainly one of the most complex functions in which the equilibrium system must interconnect inwards and outwards in order to provide a harmonious and coordinated progression of the body in the environment. Gait can be evaluated either from a clinical point of view or using sophisticated equipment. In order to investigate equilibrium and control of gait in clinical practice, the patient is asked to walk quietly in a large room to and fro first with the eyes open and then with the eyes closed. Gait with the eyes open provides generic information regarding the neurological aspects of gait. Gait with the eyes closed provides specific information regarding the equilibrium system. Not only the direction of body deviation needs to be noted but also the qualitative characteristics of gait: the width of the base of support, the position of the arms during gait, the presence of pendular synkinesias, and the stability of the head.

A simple way to evaluate equilibrium control of gait is the investigation, the patient with the eyes closed, of *stepping*, a simplified gait with the patient remaining in the same place. Generally the patient is asked to make steps for about 1 min, which is equal to about 60–80 steps. During this time, with the eyes closed, a certain forward progression of the patient is observed. The same gait characteristics can also be revealed during stepping: rotation of the stepping movement, body sway, coordination of the movement, width of base support, etc.

Technology nowadays enables sophisticated evaluation of the kinematic characteristics of single steps and the whole gait cycle to be done. The best-known equipment is based on the detection of a single marker placed on a specific point of the lower limbs: the ankle, the knee, the pelvis, etc. The ELITE (BTS, Milan) system is an example of this type of equipment. Markers are passive hemispheres that are lit by an infrared flash. Four videocameras film the patient and the markers. A computer records the televized images and frame by frame it follows the markers and sends the information to the software, which calculates the displacement of the markers with respect to time and with respect to each other (Fig. 3.12A). Another type of equipment is the CMS 70P system (Zebris, Tubingen), which consists of a measuring sensor with integrated evaluation electronics and stand, and a PC plug-in card. The measuring procedure is based on the exact determination of the three-dimensional position of the small ultrasound transmitters used as markers, by measurement of the sound pulse time. The measuring system operates up to a distance of 2 m. The markers are attached in a standard manner by means of adhesive patches to the hip, knee, ankle and ball of the foot, on both sides of the body. To determine the gait phases, thin foot contact switches are stuck to the heel and the ball of the foot. The left and the right side of the body are measured in succession. After the interactive selection of the time segments to be analyzed, a report is automatically prepared. Here, angles of the joints, the foot rotation and the lateral movements of the extremities are presented as time-dependent curves and as maximum values. The individual gait phases, the step length, the cadence and the average speed are evaluated. Information about instabilities is obtained from the averaged and normalized curves of all the individual steps and their standard deviations.

Both systems can be equipped with analog channels for simultaneous determination of EMG or force platform data. A surface telemetric EMG (Fig. 3.12B) device provides information regarding the activation and the sequence of contraction of the main muscles involved: hamstring, gastrocnemius, tibialis, etc. The systems are then completed by a force platform that reveals the reaction of the ground during stepping. A computer evaluates the displacement of each marker, and thus of each leg segment, during a single step and thus the temporal relationship between the activation of a muscle and displacement of a body segment.

A simple way to evaluate gait function with special regard to equilibrium function is the instrumental investigation of stepping. The specific method is *craniocorpography* (CCG), developed by C. F. Claussen. It has proved to be one of the most efficient, quick, objective and quantitative tests for screening equilibrium function for nearly 20 years. The West German Labour Security Surveillance Board officially introduced it for occupational medical ability testing in 1983.

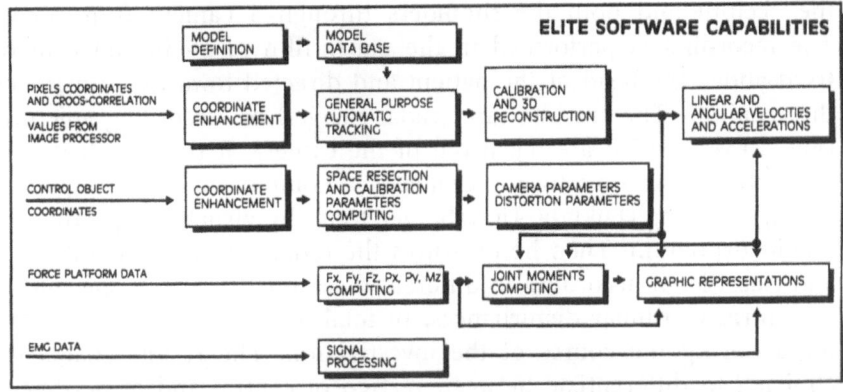

A

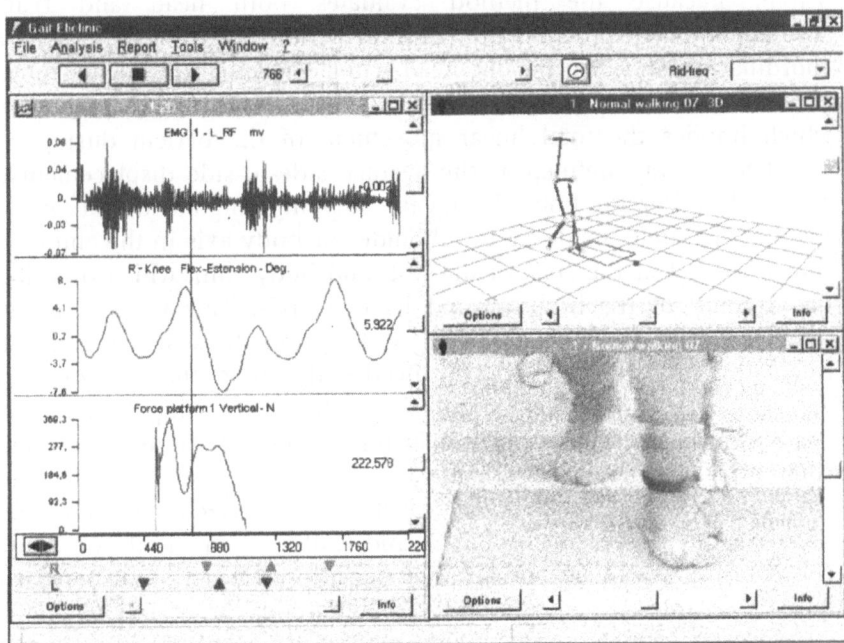

B

Fig. 3.12. A Organization of the ELITE technology. **B** Example of ELITE recording with contemporary EMG and force plate reaction recordings

CCG records the light tracings from light bulbs on the forehead, the occiput and both the shoulders through a camera from above. The recording is performed in the paper film of an instant camera, fixed above the head of the patient and directed towards a mirror on the ceiling. The results are radar-image-like recording pictures (Fig. 3.13A), which are taken out of the camera at the end of the investigation. The investigator evaluates a complete movement pattern during stepping (Fukuda, Unterberger tests) by visually inspecting the craniocorpogram. Then he measures the radar-image-like photograph and classifies it according to different disease patterns, i.e., peripheral or central vestibular disturbances. In total four parameters are monitored during the course of the investigation. The results enable the clinician to differentiate between vertigo of central and of peripheral origin. Because the method evaluates both head and trunk (shoulders), CCG provides unique information regarding both general coordination and, specifically, head-trunk coordination during movement. The CCG parameters (Fig. 3.13B) are: linear displacement, which implies the total linear movement of the patient during the test; lateral sway, defined as the average side-to-side displacement of the head and/or the body during the stepping; angular deviation, defined as the angle made by the shoulder or body axis in the end position with that at the start of the test; and body spin, which describes the rotation of the body around its own axis. This value is always found to correlate with the angular deviation. It is also possible to calculate in the rest position the head-body angle, the torticollis angle, which provides information about the relationship between the head and trunk either at rest or during movement. Figure 3.14 shows some typical abnormal CCG patterns.

Craniocorpography has been recently computerized using the technology implemented in the ELITE and CMS systems. Both the digital computerized CCG systems provide specific information also regarding stance and static posture. Thus digital CCG is a complement of stabilometry, which provides information on head-trunk reciprocal stabilization in the upright position. CMS-CCG measures the positions in space of four ultrasound transmitters (markers); two of them define the position of the head, and the other two define the position of the shoulders (Fig. 3.15). The ultrasonic pulses emitted by the markers are received by microphones in the measuring sensor. The position of the markers is calculated by timing the interval between emission and reception of the ultrasonic pulses. This allows the marker movements to be represented in transversal projection and further characteristic quantities to be established. In Fig. 3.15 the preparation

Fig. 3.13. A Typical normal craniocorpogram. **B** Parameters of craniocorpography

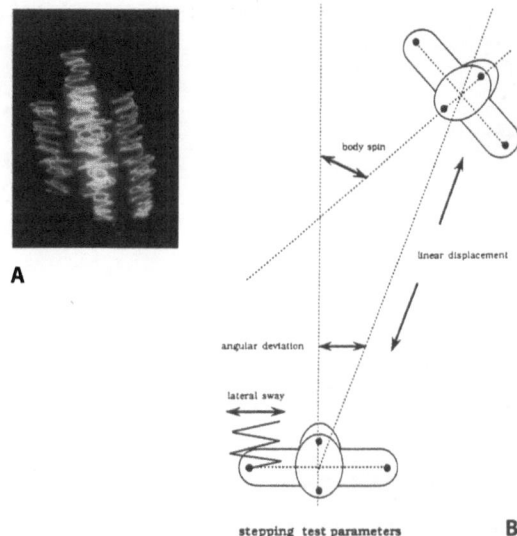

A

body spin

linear displacement

angular deviation

lateral sway

stepping test parameters

B

Fig. 3.14A–F. Examples of craniocorpograms. **A** Normal; **B** peripheral extralabyrinthine deficit; **C** vestibular deficit; **D** lower limb propioceptive deficit; **E** central deficit; **F** mixed peripheral-central vestibular deficit

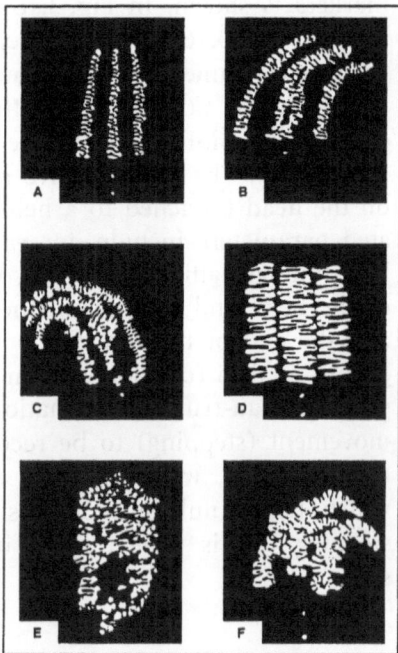

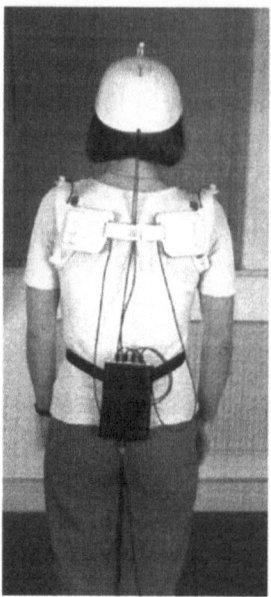

Fig. 3.15. Preparation of the patient for CMS-CCG

of the patient using a helmet for the head markers and the shoulder markers is shown. In Fig. 3.16 A a typical stance test is represented, while in Fig. 3.16B a typical stepping, dynamic pattern is shown. The evaluated parameters are the same as for traditional CCG.

The *digital CCG* based on the ELITE technology has been developed at the BioEngineering Center of the Don Gnocchi Foundation, Milan, Italy. The same passive markers have been used, placing them on the head (attached to a helmet) and on the shoulders. The evaluated parameters include, for each marker: lateral sway and velocity, longitudinal path and velocity, total distance, mean velocity, rotation of the head and rotation of the shoulders, comparing the beginning and the end of the test and body spin. The comparison of the four groups of data (one for each marker) enables precise information regarding head-trunk coordination either during the stance or during movement (stepping) to be recorded. In Fig. 3.17 a normal standing test is shown, while Fig. 3.18 shows an abnormal standing test in which head/trunk sway is easily detectable. In Fig. 3.19 a normal stepping test is shown while in Fig. 3.20 a pathological pattern is seen.

Fig. 3.16. Examples of stance results (**A**) and stepping findings (**B**) during computerized recording of ultrasound CCG

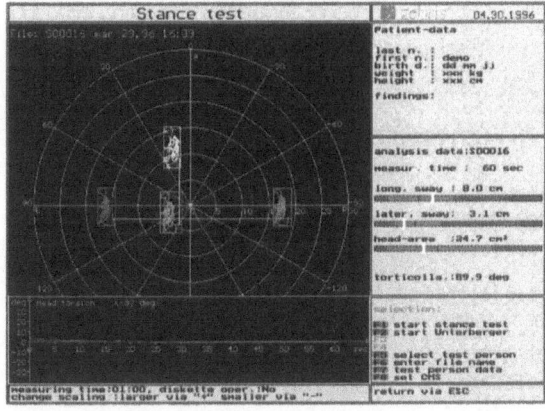

A

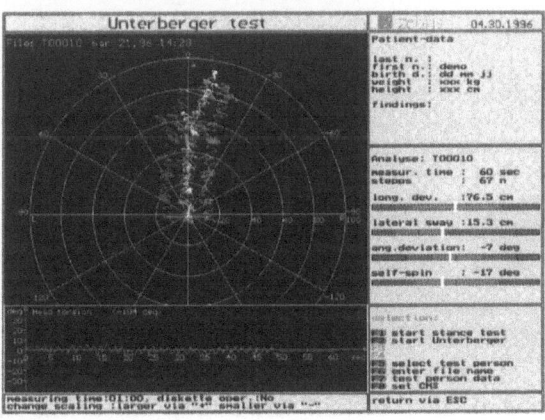

B

3.4 Specific Approach: Orientation

The evaluation of orientation aspects concerns the cognitive aspects of the equilibrium function. Visuoconstructive functions can be investigated using the Bender Gestalt visuomotor test, which is fast (15 min) and simple to perform for both the clinician and the patient. The patient has to copy as well as possible nine geometric paintings. The modality of the copies is evaluated according to the Pascal-Suttel method. The aim of the test is to evaluate and quantify emotional disturbances.

Orientation is simply evaluated in a clinical manner. The basic tests are the classical so-called cerebellar tests: the index-nose, the index-knee and the heel-knee tests. Although they are considered tests for

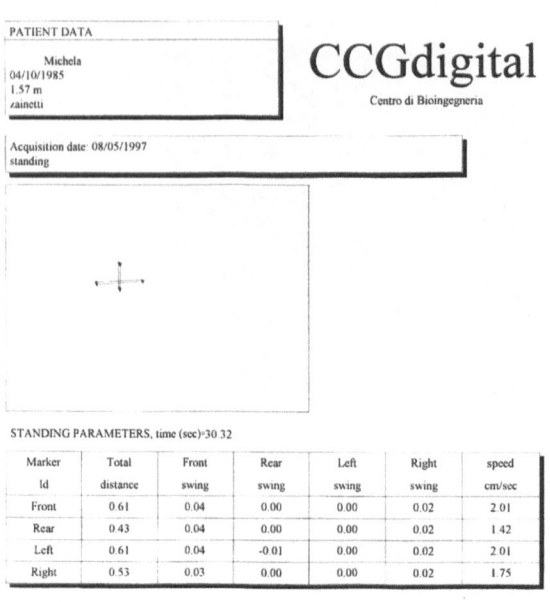

Fig. 3.17. Normal standing test during recording of digital CCG

STANDING PARAMETERS, time (sec):30.32

Marker Id	Total distance	Front swing	Rear swing	Left swing	Right swing	speed cm/sec
Front	0.61	0.04	0.00	0.00	0.02	2.01
Rear	0.43	0.04	0.00	0.00	0.02	1.42
Left	0.61	0.04	-0.01	0.00	0.02	2.01
Right	0.53	0.03	0.00	0.00	0.02	1.75

Rotation	Starting	Ending	Difference	Spin body
Shoulder	-2°	-3°	-1°	
Neck	2°	3°	1°	180°

cerebellar function, these simple tests investigate the capability of the subject to recognize the reciprocal position of different body segments; in a certain sense they reflect the inner representation of the body schema (inner orientation).

The internal representation of posture may be clinically investigated in a simple manner. In the supine position the patient is correctly aligned along a longitudinal axis, with eyes open. The eyes are then closed and the clinician moves the head from time to time, placing it in a lateral, first rightward, then leftward, position. The patient has to reposition his head correctly, with the eyes closed. In this way it is possible to evaluate whether the patient possesses a correct sense of alignment of the head-trunk or if he places his head in a lateral position. Other simple subjective vertical and horizontal parameters may be investigated, with the sitting patient asked, with eyes closed, to put a pen vertically straight in front of his nose (subjective vertical) and horizontally straight in front of his eyes (subjective horizontal).

Fig. 3.18. Abnormal
standing test

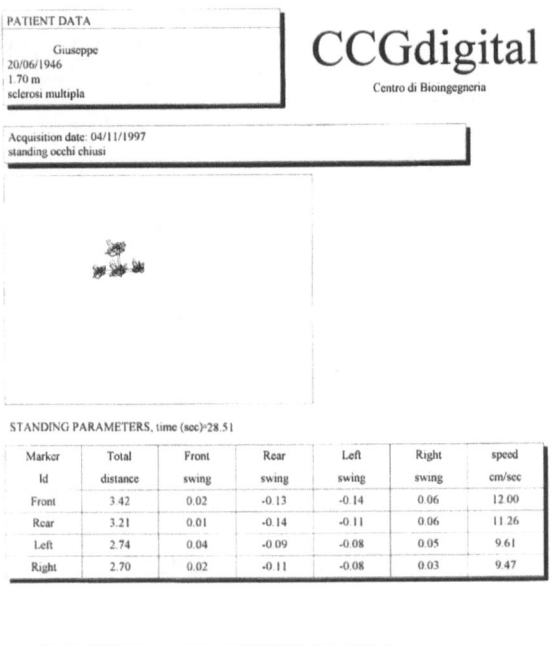

PATIENT DATA

Giuseppe
20/06/1946
1.70 m
sclerosi multipla

CCGdigital

Centro di Bioingegneria

Acquisition date: 04/11/1997
standing occhi chiusi

STANDING PARAMETERS, time (sec)=28.51

Marker	Total	Front	Rear	Left	Right	speed
Id	distance	swing	swing	swing	swing	cm/sec
Front	3.42	0.02	-0.13	-0.14	0.06	12.00
Rear	3.21	0.01	-0.14	-0.11	0.06	11.26
Left	2.74	0.04	-0.09	-0.08	0.05	9.61
Right	2.70	0.02	-0.11	-0.08	0.03	9.47

Rotation	Starting	Ending	Difference	Spin body
Shoulder	-5°	-2°	3°	
Neck	1°	-3°	-4°	-1°

Assessment of the *visual subjective vertical* in which subjects have to place a line vertical in an otherwise totally darkened room is sensitive to acute peripheral or central deficits. The semicircular canal and visual or proprioceptive stimuli induce profound modifications of the settings of the visual vertical in normal subjects. The simplicity of the procedure, the inexpensive techniques involved and the clear abnormalities in some cases make this technique an attractive one for the clinician.

CCG allows the documentation of a particular aspect of orientation, spatial orientation in the environment. The patient is asked to stand with eyes closed (better if blindfolded). Then the examiner, without any previous explanation to the patient about the modality and the finality of the test, gives the patient some simple commands:

1. One step forward.
2. Another step forward.
3. Turn rightwards 90°.
4. Two steps forward.
5. Turns rightwards 90°.
6. One step forward.

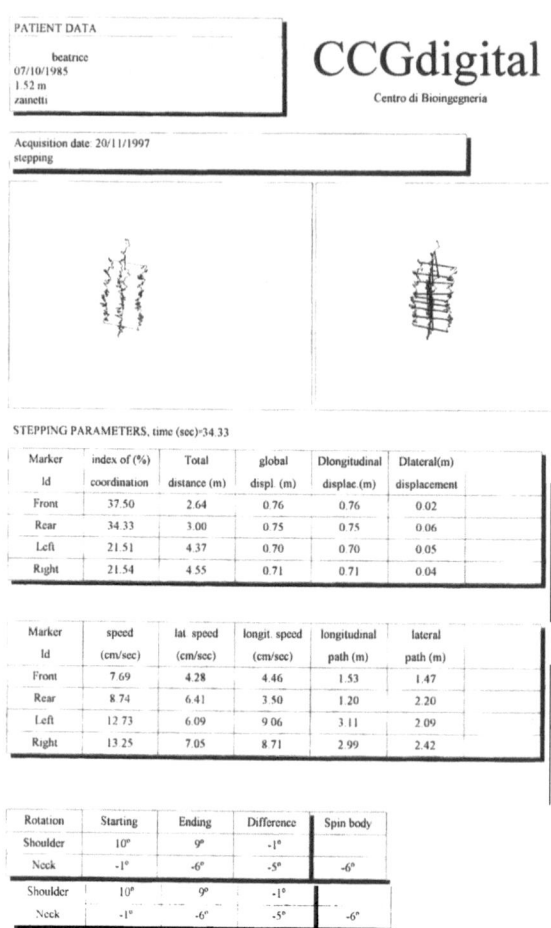

Fig. 3.19. Normal stepping dCCG findings

STEPPING PARAMETERS, time (sec)=34.33

Marker Id	index of (%) coordination	Total distance (m)	global displ. (m)	Dlongitudinal displac.(m)	Dlateral(m) displacement
Front	37.50	2.64	0.76	0.76	0.02
Rear	34.33	3.00	0.75	0.75	0.06
Left	21.51	4.37	0.70	0.70	0.05
Right	21.54	4.55	0.71	0.71	0.04

Marker Id	speed (cm/sec)	lat. speed (cm/sec)	longit. speed (cm/sec)	longitudinal path (m)	lateral path (m)
Front	7.69	4.28	4.46	1.53	1.47
Rear	8.74	6.41	3.50	1.20	2.20
Left	12.73	6.09	9.06	3.11	2.09
Right	13.25	7.05	8.71	2.99	2.42

Rotation	Starting	Ending	Difference	Spin body
Shoulder	10°	9°	-1°	
Neck	-1°	-6°	-5°	-6°
Shoulder	10°	9°	-1°	
Neck	-1°	-6°	-5°	-6°

7. One step forward.

8. Now return to the starting position.

The real orientation test is the prompt No. 8: the patient must have in his mind his path and on the basis of this simple spatial orientation might be able to recognize his new position and be able to reach the starting position. At the end of the test the patient is asked to draw his path on a sheet of paper. In this way all the processes that lead to orientation in an environment can be evaluated: the skill of recognizing the position in the environment and the skill of reconstructing and of reproducing a motion experience. CCG allows the test to be documented. In Fig. 3.21 a normal pattern is shown. The patient was also able to draw correctly the path performed. The patient in Fig. 3.22 was neither able to complete the path nor to reproduce it.

Fig. 3.20. Pathological stepping dCGG findings

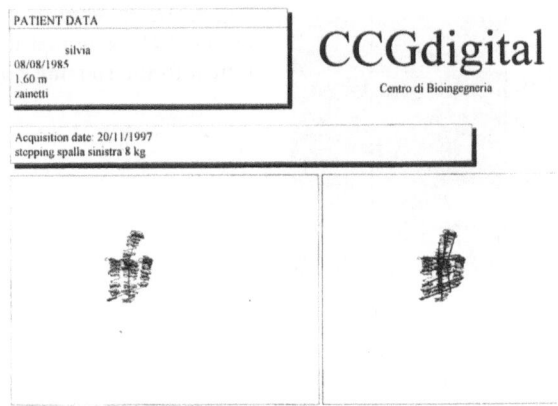

PATIENT DATA

silvia
08/08/1985
1.60 m
zanetti

CCGdigital

Centro di Bioingegneria

Acquisition date: 20/11/1997
stepping spalla sinistra 8 kg

STEPPING PARAMETERS, time (sec)=30.54

Marker Id	index of (%) coordination	Total distance (m)	global displ. (m)	Dlongitudinal displac.(m)	Dlateral(m) displacement	
Front	16.53	6.11	0.34	0.34	0.08	
Rear	16.62	6.92	0.38	0.38	-0.01	
Left	15.79	5.70	0.38	0.38	-0.01	
Right	15.75	5.27	0.24	0.24	0.00	

Marker Id	speed (cm/sec)	lat. speed (cm/sec)	longit. speed (cm/sec)	longitudinal path (m)	lateral path (m)	
Front	20.01	18.04	5.17	1.58	5.51	
Rear	22.66	20.40	5.86	1.79	6.23	
Left	18.67	15.26	6.91	2.11	4.66	
Right	17.26	13.72	7.04	2.15	4.19	

Rotation	Starting	Ending	Difference	Spin body
Shoulder	-20°	1°	21°	
Neck	19°	15°	-4°	17°

Fig. 3.21. Normal orientation test recorded with C-CG (**A**) and the drawings made by the patient (**B**)

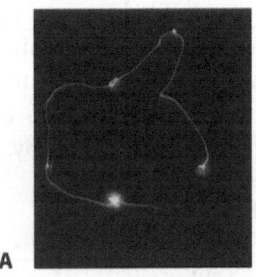

A

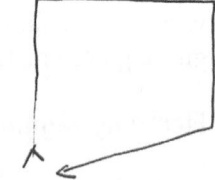

B

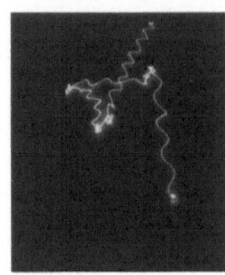

Fig. 3.22A, B. Abnormal orientation test. **A** and **B** as in Fig. 3.21. Note that the patient is neither able to return to the starting position nor to draw the path

A

B

3.5 Using Complex Vestibular Tests To Investigate the Resources of Diseased Equilibrium Function

C.-F. CLAUSSEN

Introduction

The equilibrium function is regulated on several sensory input stations as well as on several different brain levels. The complex equilibrium regulating the system also inherits a broad spectrum of regulatory plasticity. Modern equilibriometry is a noninvasive method of investigation that allows the establishment of a neuro-otological topo-diagnostic scheme, which can be used for a correlated therapy of the various dysequilibrium states. It can also be used for monitoring and guiding systematic antivertiginous therapy.

Electronystagmography

Of the wide variety of equilibriometric investigations, the electronystagmographically recorded caloric nystagmus has proved to be the most important clinical tool in neuro-otology. In 1906, Barany described the caloric nystagmus provoked by syringing warm and cold water into the external ear and Ruttin (1922) released the caloric nystagmus by gas insufflation to the external ear. In 1942 Fitzgerald and Hallpike introduced a quantitative caloric nystagmus time duration scale for the bithermally released monaural vestibular ocular nystagmus. To measure the nystagmus duration, they used Frenzel's glasses and a stopwatch.

In 1922, Schott invented electronystagmography (ENG) in Cologne, but it was only in 1956 that Henriksson systematically utilized ENG by means of the ENG derivation of the slow caloric nystagmus component to demonstrate the postcaloric nystagmus by means of a recorded bell-shaped nystagmus distribution on a plot with a slow paper speed. Torok began nystagmus frequency analysis in 1948, and in 1957 he used a frequency analysis of the postcaloric nystagmus during the culmination phenomenon in a distribution of the postcaloric nystagmus reaction similar to the Henriksson technique for establishing a quantitative response analysis.

Since its invention by Schott in 1922, ENG has provided neuro-otology with a universal instrument for noninvasively recording eye movements with eyes open or closed, during wakefulness or sleep, in the resting or moving positions, which can easily can be submitted to A/D conversion for use in diagnostic computer systems.

The procedure we have used in our neuro-otologic laboratories for 30 years is to record, using a set of skin electrodes in orthogonal positions around both eyes (Fig. 3.23), the eye movements both horizon-

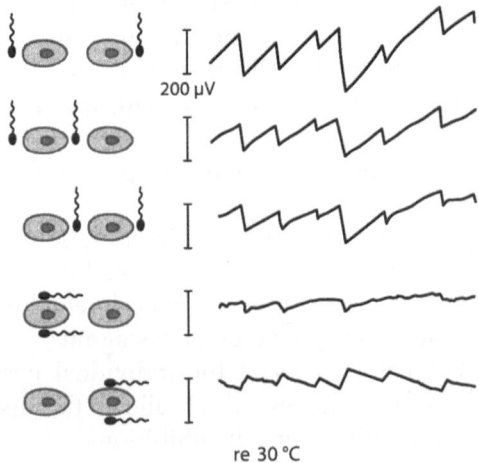

Fig. 3.23. The ENG traces are placed in the following order on the recorder strip chart: *Trace 1,* recording of the electrical movements in the horizontal plane of both eyes; *trace 2,* horizontal recording from the right eye; *trace 3,* horizontal recording from the left eye; *trace 4,* vertical recording from the right eye; *trace 5,* vertical recording from the left eye

tally and vertically on an eight-channel polygraph on five traces, together with an electrocardiogram on three channels. The ECG is a very suitable method for documenting the vestibulovegetative reactions for nausea analysis. The nystagmus potentials are usually between 40 and 100 µV per beat.

The Caloric Butterfly Test

As the caloric nystagmus test is the most significant neuro-otological test procedure in the field of equilibriometry, it must be carefully prepared, performed and evaluated. The caloric test is performed according to the butterfly scheme of Claussen. The patient lies in the supine position with rinsing catheters inserted into his external ear meatuses and water-recollecting bags attached to his auricles. Twenty milliliters of water at either 30 °C or 44 °C is injected through the catheter in 30 s. From the start of rinsing up to 180 s the test is recorded electronystagmographically with a five-channel ENG technique to record the ENG in the horizontal plane both binocularly and monocularly and to record the eye movements in the vertical plane monocularly on both eyes (Fig. 3.23). During the final phase of the electronystagmogram the nystagmus beats are identified, counted and transferred to the typical butterfly chart of Claussen.

After the conversion of the four raw caloric ENGs into a synoptic test chart, the Claussen butterfly chart (Fig. 3.24) is drawn, which provides the investigator with the following four items of quantitative information:

1. A comparison of the responses from both ears, with left or right ear inhibition.
2. The nystagmus beat direction compared with central nystagmus inhibition or central directional nystagmus preponderance.
3. A comparison of the experimental nystagmus intensity with the underlying spontaneous nystagmus.
4. A comparison of the individual nystagmus reactions with external normal ranges, which allows the discrimination between reactional inhibitions and disinhibitions.

Topodiagnostic relations have been established on the basis of animal experiments with destruction of typical vestibular ocular pathway structures. We have also evaluated pathway lesions in postmortem material. Finally we have evaluated the morphological diagnostics of a large body of clinical material using X-rays, arteriography, CT scans

Fig. 3.24. Claussen's butterfly chart

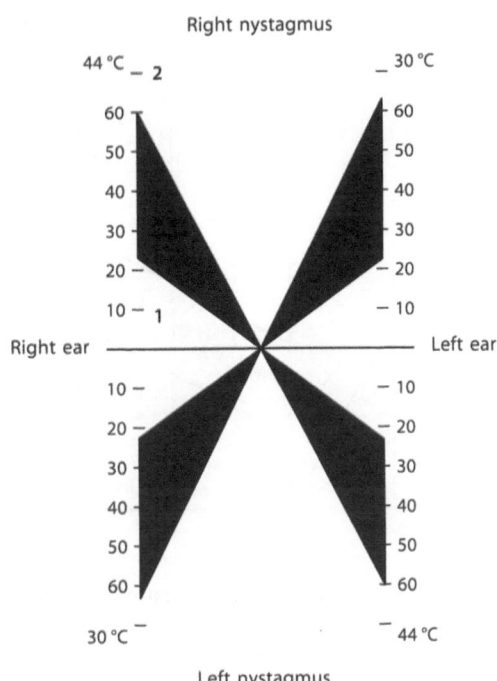

and MRI scans. Thus our functional test results have also been correlated with lesions in morphological structures.

The Rotatory Intensity Damping Test

Rotatory nystagmus tests use a binaural stimulus technique. The Rotatory Intensity Damping Test (RIDT), which has been used by our group for more than 20 years, combines a supraliminal steplike perrotatory stimulus with a supramaximal needle-shaped postrotatory stimulus in a trapezoidal stimulus pattern. The per- and postrotatory nystagmus results are evaluated similarly to the butterfly characteristics. They are jointly represented using an "L-chart." The left segment exhibits the perrotatory and the right the postrotatory nystagmus responses with respect to the normal ranges (see Fig. 3.25).

The RIDT is performed on the electronically regulated rotatory chair with linear acceleration and velocity patterns. During a perrotatory phase at $3°/s^2$ for a duration of 30 s, the patient is linearly accelerated from 0 to $90°/s$. Then for a period of 180 s the chair rotates constantly at $90°/s$. After 210 s from the onset of the test, a break is

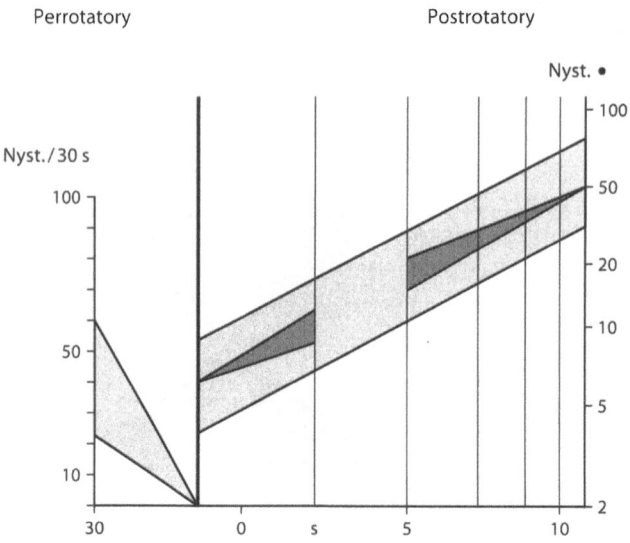

Fig. 3.25. "L"-scheme of the Rotatory Intensity Damping Test (RIDT)

inserted within 1/3 s to bring the chair to a standstill, which means an accelerative force of $270°/s^2$. Throughout this time the nystagmus beats are recorded with the same ENG scheme applied during the caloric test. The nystagmus beats are evaluated during the perrotatory part of the test in an analogous way to the caloric test. During the culmination phase the nystagmus beats are identified over 30 s. The intensity is transferred into a characteristic pattern in the L-chart scheme. The postrotatory stimulus delivers an e-function type of nystagmus response to a needle-shaped stimulus. This response must be handled in a different way. The damping function pattern therefore is shown in the L-chart scheme on a double logarithmic scale.

Perrotatory tracings show three broad patterns of behavior. Either the response lies within normal limits, or it may be inhibited or overactive. Inhibition during rotation, however, has a different clinical significance than caloric inhibition, as it may mean both a central and a peripheral lesion. Statistically, the incidence of inhibition in the RIDT is far greater than in the butterfly chart. The perrotatory results should be compared with the ipsilateral warm caloric responses. Discrepancies in both these tests indicate a *vestibular recruitment* or *decruitment,* thus reflecting the severity of the pathology concerned. The postrotatory test has proved to be of major clinical significance in children, where the responses are markedly dampened. Furthermore, supratentorial lesions are seen to produce changes in this value, especially in the gradient of the response.

Complex Nystagmus-Based Equilibrium Reactions

Vestibular Stimulus Response Intensity Comparison

Vestibular Stimulus Response Intensity Comparisons (VSRIC) leading to the definition of vestibular recruitment can be achieved using intensity-graded supraliminal stimuli of two different pairs:
1. Small and major monolateral caloric stimuli at the same temperature, cold or warm components.
2. Small and major bilateral perrotatory stimuli of the same directional component, right or left, or
3. A monolateral caloric stimulus of the same directional component used as the weaker trigger combined with a stronger bilateral perrotatory stimulus of the same directional component used as the stronger supraliminal stimulus.

The third mode has proved to be clinically most efficient as it only needs to evaluate the already existing nystagmus data from the caloric butterfly and the perrotatory nystagmus of the RIDT in the VSRIC.

It is well known that the caloric stimulus falls into the type of a ramp-shaped supraliminal stimulus. The perrotatory stimulus, however, is a step-shaped supraliminal stimulus. Additionally the caloric stimulus is applied monaurally whereas the perrotatory stimulus acts binaurally upon the semicircular canals. Thus the caloric stimulus can easily be detected as the weaker stimulus and the perrotatory stimulus as the stronger one. When recording ipsidirectional stimulus results such as the right ear warm nystagmus and the perrotatory right nystagmus, the test characteristics can be compared with the underlying normal ranges (caloric butterfly warm segments and ipsilateral perrotatory RIDT segments) with respect to their activity categories.

There are three typical categories of behavior. Either the two test responses fall equally in the normal ranges, which is *parallel* normal behavior, or the responses are inhibited or disinhibited in parallel (Fig. 3.26, top left). The second category is the *recruiting phenomenon.* Either the caloric test is inhibited and the perrotatory ipsidirectional nystagmus is normal or disinhibited (Fig. 3.26, top right) or the caloric stimulus lies in the normal range and the perrotatory stimulus is disinhibited. Only the first of these three patterns, which is mainly an inhibition of the weaker caloric stimulus with respect to the normal reaction of the stronger perrotatory nystagmus, holds for

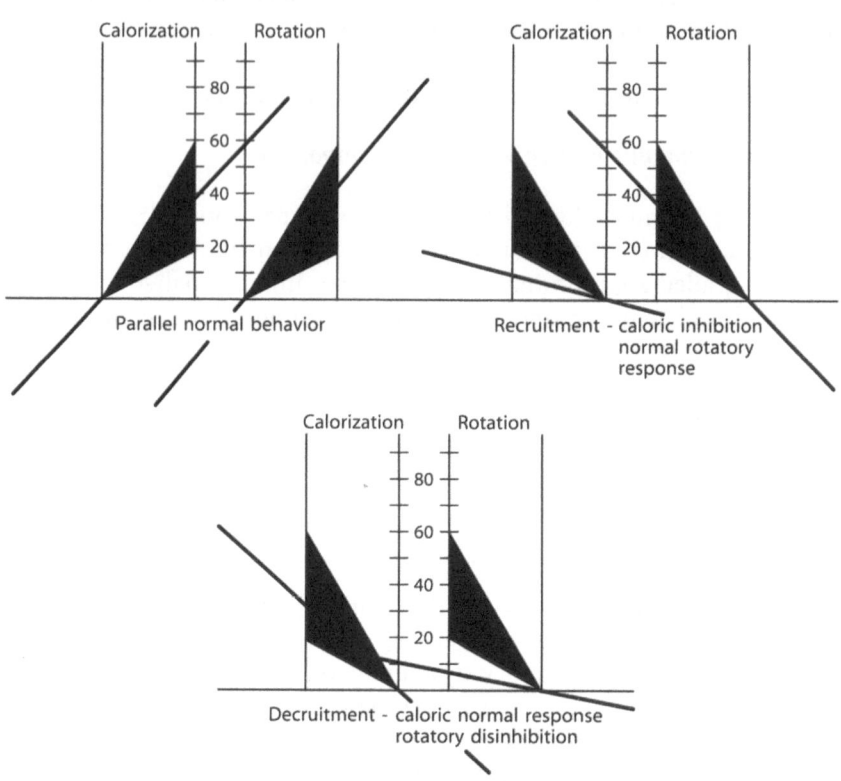

Fig. 3.26. Scheme of three fundamental types of VSRIC: a parallel normal behavior, a recruiting phenomenon and a decruiting phenomenon (caloric butterfly warm segments, *left*, and ipsilateral perrotatory RIDT segments, *right*)

a recruitment phenomenon of the peripheral vestibular type. On increasing the stimulus force this vestibular equilibrium system then becomes recruiting. However, if the weaker stimulus lies in normal ranges and the stronger stimulus evokes a response pattern of the disinhibited type, we are facing a hidden central nystagmus disinhibition. This is commonly seen in disorders such as vertebrobasilar insufficiency. The third recruitment pattern, which is rare, shows a peripheral blockage type of the caloric warm response, while at the same time, however, extreme central disinhibition. These patterns are mainly found in cerebellopontine angle lesions and more frequently in those of the vascular than of the acoustic neurinoma type.

The third group of vestibular stimulus response intensity comparison patterns (Fig. 3.26, bottom) always has a higher response intensity in the weaker stimulus responses to the calorics than to the stronger of the rotatory stimuli. Either the caloric test result is normal and the perrotatory test is inhibited or the caloric test result is disinhibited and the perrotatory test is inhibited or normal. This pattern is called vestibular *recruitment,* which demonstrates a central nystagmus generator blockage for a higher load of stimulus force.

Calorization Pendulum Interference Test

The calorization pendulum interference test (CPIT) combines the ocular vertical light pendulum tracking test with the monaural calorically induced horizontal nystagmus test. To obtain the typical visual interference as a quantitative measurement in a first trial, a conventional caloric test is performed. The test results are synoptically charted by means of the Claussen butterfly chart. Then in a second step the lateral vestibular canal and the visual system are brought at the same time into spatial interference of the two receptors. The test result is a modified nystagmus signal due to visual vestibular interaction. The patient is requested to follow the vertically swinging pendulum with a smooth ocular up and downward pursuit. At the same time a calorically induced nystagmus is monaurally provoked at $30\,°C$ or $44\,°C$ with 20 ml water during 30 s rinsing time. The ocular eye movements are recorded by means of a five-channel polygraphic ENG scheme from 40 s to 120 s after the onset of the calorization.

The result of the CPIT is plotted as for the pure caloric test in the butterfly scheme. The pendulum tracking movement can either suppress the caloric nystagmus or trigger it similarly to a disinhibition. Thus, clinically hidden inhibitory brainstem nystagmus dysfunctions can be unveiled by this test.

In a study of 129 neuro-otological patients between the age of 10 years and 70 years, who underwent the CPIT, 59 (45.74%) were male and 70 (54.26%) were female. All the patients performed the same scheme of investigations with an initial pure caloric test with butterfly evaluation followed by a caloric test with eyes open gazing at the vertically swinging pendulum at 0.3 cps oscillation frequency. The nystagmus beat rate during the 30 s of the culmination period was measured, thus delivering the central nystagmus frequency as the beat rate during 30 s. The center of the culmination window exhibits the culmination latency in seconds from the onset of the calorization.

The data for these test results are shown in Tables 3.4 and 3.5. From this overview we conclude that the calorically induced nystagmus is depressed during vertical ocular pursuit with respect to the

Table 3.4. Caloric nystagmus frequencies during 30 s of culmination without and with ocular tracking in 129 neuro-otological patients

Parameter	Without ocular tracking mean	Standard deviation	With ocular tracking mean	Standard deviation
Right, 44 °C	37.9	17.9	27.1	19.7
Right, 30 °C	43.8	17.6	30.6	19.8
Left, 44 °C	41.8	19.6	27.3	18.6
Left, 30 °C	48.3	19.8	35.8	21.1

Table 3.5. Culmination latency of the calorically induced nystagmus without and with simultaneously vertical ocular tracking

Parameter	Without vertical ocular tracking (mean)	Standard deviation	With vertical ocular tracking (mean)	Standard deviation
Right, 44 °C	71.1	17.3	56.8	22.8
Right, 30 °C	64.9	16.3	60.0	19.9
Left, 44 °C	68.5	18.6	61.6	18.9
Left, 30 °C	70.9	19.7	62.5	15.3

central nystagmus frequency of the butterfly as well as shortened with respect to the culmination latency.

The results of the CPIT show that the vestibular system, the optomotor system and the retino-ocular system are acting together in an overlapped and interinjected manner. From other experiments of ocular fixation indexes and retino-ocular movement analysis, we know that there is a strong dampening factor through especially the retinal input in various planes of movement upon the vestibular ocular reflex arch. However, our cases not only exhibit the pattern of reduced activity due to vestibular stimulation, but in special cases also the opposite. Especially in brainstem disorders due to atherosclerosis, diabetes mellitus, postconcussional states, etc., frequently disinhibit. Thus we can also clinically demonstrate by means of the spatial stimulus interference that there exists a labile trend for brainstem disintegration in central equilibrium control, which may lead to vertigo attacks in everyday life.

Caloric Adaptation Cyclogram

For temporal stimulus interference testing, it is supposed that a memory (copy) of earlier stimuli is influencing successive reactions. Thus, phenomena like learning or habituation can be induced. Temporal stimulus interference is being tested by means of the caloric adaptation cyclogram (CAC).

For testing by means of the caloric adaptation cyclogram, we use a series of ten consecutive caloric tests with electronystagmographic ocular nystagmus recordings. The maximum frequency responses during the final phase are successively transferred into butterfly characteristics. The calorizations always use the same modality. Thus, either a warm or a cold test of the same ear is repeated ten times. Then, by means of a mobile butterfly chart system, we start to rotate the quadrants so that every successive characteristic is established on the characteristic prior to the last one as a baseline. Thus we induce the skeleton of a coil, which either remains in circular shape, spinning towards the center, or spinning off the center. Especially those candidates who demonstrate a spin towards the center in the chart of the caloric adaptation cyclogram exhibit a well-established capacity for learning from successive monaural caloric vestibular stimuli, which gives them a good prognosis for stress control after vestibular losses.

Discussion

The human equilibrium system derives much of its strength and plasticity from the fact that specific neuronal and growing software is molded in childhood during its maturation phase under the influence of permanent information from the terrestrial world in which we live. The human software overlying the structural, sensorial and central nervous anatomical hardware creates the so-called space concept within the midbrain. The sensorial equilibrium tetrade comprises: (a) the visual receptors of the retina, (b) the inertia receptors in the vestibular systems, (c) the proprioceptive receptors in the muscles, tendons and joints of the kinesthetic perception and (d) the cochlea receptors for spatial sound perception. The integration is mainly performed within the brainstem and especially in the midbrain. However, there are also contributions from supratentorial centers around the posterior part of the upper temporal lobe gyrus as well as from the basal ganglia and the cerebellum. Projections from corrective equilibrium regulation are to be found on the motor level at the eye (nystagmus) and the motor body positioning of head, trunk and limbs. We also find responses of the vegetative type (nausea) as well as of the psychophysic type (vertigo). Regulatory changes due to equilibrium responses are also seen at the level of biochemical blood composition as well as of metabolic processes.

Equilibrium regulation, as it exists in the human, is a very complex process. Thus, failures of both sensory inputs and central equilibrium regulation may lead to various expressions of illness such as vertigo, nausea and vomitus, blurred vision, nystagmus, head and body instability, changes in cardiac rhythm, and metabolic alterations.

Facing such a broad spectrum of pathological responses, inherent in the system are many possibilities for internal stabilization and compensation. With respect to the reparation processes, we can discriminate restitution, adaptation, suppression, habituation, and compensation.

Restitution

Restitution can be defined as complete reparation after a temporally limited lesion. For instance, after an inner ear infection with severe vertigo attacks, we observe in later investigations a complete recovery of all the measurable functions, as a result of the anti-inflammatory and anti-infectious therapy. The patient then is cured and completely free from any further subjective complaints.

Adaptation

Adaptation means that the human equilibrium system can adapt itself to physiologically and pathologically altered conditions. For instance, during the process of peripheral vestibular lesions of one side we observe that the sensitivity of the opposite vestibular receptor is counterregulated through a feedback loop so that it nearly suits the condition of leveled comparisons between both the inner ears. In the follow-ups during a monolateral peripheral vestibular loss we observe an opposite side depression in the caloric butterfly and a spontaneous nystagmus beating towards the lesion (Stenger's Erholungs nystagmus). Thus, the functional adaptation after a severe peripheral vestibular lesion can precede the process of restitution.

Suppression

As mentioned above, the central regulatory system can alter the sensitivity of the vestibular, the retinal and other receptors for equilibrium regulation. In the case of an adaptation situation, we have also observed an extreme condition of this type of regulation, which we have called "vestibular suppression." In the case of vestibular suppression, we find that the central regulation suppresses complete lines of, for instance, ocular movement control in favor of the unaltered tracts, as can be proved by the calorization pendulum interference test. The regulation pattern of "suppression" sometimes also appears like a selective switch from one system to another.

Habituation

A compensation phenomenon, which includes a special learning program for movements or spatial situations, is called habituation. This is defined by the reduction of the intensity and duration of the subjective vestibular reactions such as vertigo and nausea in the case of seasickness, as well as in the correction of dys- or overreactions of the sensory motor type with a nystagmus or head and body instability. In 1906, Abels described the reduction of seasickness during long-term exposure on a boat to the habituation of the vestibular system. Bárány described functional reductions in ballet dancers, especially with respect to the decrease in the postrotatory nystagmus.

This learned reduction or blockage of physiological equilibrium reactions has to be stored in the central nervous system. It can also be forgotten if it has not been used sufficiently for a while. The habituation is not completely specific for one single vestibular stimulus, but can also be transferred from one type of stimulus to another. Therefore we have designed the cyclogram of habituation as a vestibular test model. Habituation is also possible for optokinetic stimulus modalities. In many vertigo rehabilitation programs, habituation is the goal for compensatory recovery.

Compensation

The term "compensation" describes another type of central nervous counterregulation against a functional deterioration through a vestibular or other equilibrium lesion. It utilizes supplementary functions, which are added so that an overlay of additionally activated functions covers the underlying equilibrium lesion by means of its neuronal plasticity. However, the primary lesion continues to exist and in the case of a particular conflict it can resurface in the clinical phenomenology. By means of an intermediate neuronal plasticity on the level of the vestibular nuclei, a peripheral vestibular lesion, for instance, which is primarily visible in the monolateral caloric inhibition in the butterfly calorigram as well as in the deviation towards the side of the lesion in the step-test craniocorpogram, after a while can only be continuously verified in the calorigram. However, the craniocorpography of the vestibular spinal step-test movement develops towards a regular normal picture without any further deviation, neither towards the right nor to the left, and without any pathology in the CCG sway patterns.

The question of equilibrium compensation after various types of dysequilibrium states is increasingly important, as we have to deal with many vertigo patients nowadays. As described above, many of our test combinations now allow us to receive dynamic outputs, which can be turned into prognostic evaluations.

All the three complex equilibriometric tests, the vestibular stimulus response intensity comparison (VSRIC), the spatial stimulus interference test (CPIT), and the temporal stimulus interference test (CAC), provide us with much information about equilibrium compensation, which can especially influence the psychotherapy as well as the physiotherapy and pharmacotherapy. The progress of restitution, adaptation, suppression, habituation and finally compensation guides the patient to recovery in both the patient's private and professional lives.

Furthermore we frequently find that patients suffering from vertigo are simply misdiagnosed, as tests are applied which do not cover the area of the particular defect in the equilibrium system. Therefore the neuro-otologist has to apply a network of neuro-otometric tests. Once the type and site of the lesion have been defined, we can also initiate adequate therapy, which will make use of the inborn self-regulating forces of compensation.

Neuro-otological functional data acquisition provides us with a network of multisensorial information about the status of our patients. Many of these tests are time consuming in their performance as well as evaluation. Therefore, the number of tests which can be applied at one time as well as the number of patients which can be investigated in one neuro-otological laboratory are limited. However, due to the aging of our population with increasing frequencies of age-related dysequilibrium states (presbyvertigo, presbyataxia, presbynausea), there is a steadily growing demand for these investigations. Therefore, it is only a question of time before we are able to facilitate the automatic evaluation and to increase the amount of information available to the investigator.

When using these tests we use the following hierarchy of efficiency, which is listed below. However, the list is not yet complete:
1. Vestibular ocular caloric test with butterfly chart evaluation.
2. Stepping and standing craniocorpography test.
3. Acoustic brainstem evoked potentials (ABEPs).
4. Optokinetic pendular tracking test.

5. Perrotatory nystagmus.
6. Vestibular stimulus response intensity comparison (VSRIC).
7. Nystagmus coordination test.
8. Visually evoked potentials (VEPs).
9. Acoustic late evoked potentials (ALEPs).
10. Postrotatory nystagmus.
11. Complex equilibriometric tests.
12. Spontaneous nystagmus.

The empirical list of the diagnostic importance of the neuro-oto-metric tests shows that the rank position of the complex equilibrio-metric tests lies in the fourth quarter of 12 tests. However, the VSRIC automatically applies when tests 1 and 5 are performed on the same patient.

The above-mentioned tests are generally used to establish a topo-diagnosis and to start and monitor the therapy of the neurosensorial dysfunctions in about 300 different neuro-otological diseases.

4 Treatment

The human equilibrium system derives much of its strength and plasticity from the fact that the specific neuronal and growing software is molded in childhood during the maturation phase, under the influence of permanent information from the world we live in. The software overlying the structural, sensorial and central nervous hardware creates the so-called space concept within the brain. Failures of sensory inputs as well as of central equilibrium regulation may lead to various expressions of illness such as vertigo, nausea and vomiting, blurred vision, nystagmus, head and body instability, changes in cardiac rhythm and metabolic alterations. The system has many inborn possibilities for internal stabilization and compensation; in fact after injury various neurophysiological phenomena are involved in the restoration of the equilibrium function. Rehabilitation specifically activates one or more of these phenomena:

Restitution can be defined as complete reparation after a temporally limited lesion.

Adaptation means that the human equilibrium system can adapt itself to physiologically, as well as to pathologically, altered conditions. The central regulatory system can alter the sensitivity of the vestibular, retinal and other receptors used to regulate equilibrium. It comprises all phenomena which ensure that a patient with a persisting peripheral dysfunctional state reattains normal – or near normal – behavior in relation to his space orientation and balance in rest as well as when executing movements. He again maintains his erect standing position and no longer has an "odd" feeling categorized as vertigo or dizziness. A number of mechanisms contribute here, acting at different levels of the central nervous system. The first definition can be applied to adaptation in the strict physiological sense: a change of response during application of a stimulus, e.g., a prolonged acceleration which brings about a response decline. Fatigue is characterized by a response decline which develops slowly. It increases with stimulus intensity and progresses indefinitely with time. Such adaptation is characterized by a response decline which develops rapidly at first and thereafter slowly, finally reaching a constant or fully adapted level. Adaptation phenomena in the same time sense are also attributed to a mechanism at the level of the cupola, which is also direction specific. The second definition fits the broader concept of adaptation. The messages sent by the sense organs into the brainstem are increasingly suppressed and prevented from reaching the higher centers the longer the steady state in the surrounding world persists. The subject has adapted to conditions imposed by the outer world. However, the slightest change in stimulatory conditions not pertaining to the steady state will cause alarm.

Habituation is defined by the reduction of the intensity and duration of the subjective vestibular reactions, for example, vertigo and nausea in the case of seasickness. Habituation is a term used in the sense that repeated exposure to a "mismatched" sensory situation (e.g., during caloric testing, postural vertigo or motion sickness conditions) induces such changes in the central processing as to annihilate the undesirable effects and to do so with a prolonged effect. It has been based upon the development of conditioned compensatory reactions to oppose inappropriate responses associated with visuovestibular conflicts and exposure to unusual motion environments. The basic characteristics of vestibular habituation, regarding oculomotor aspects, are:

- Acquisition, which is manifested by a progressive decline in VOR response during the period of stimulation.
- Retention, which is manifested by the persistence of a modified VOR response after a period of rest. It is cumulative and long-lasting.
- Certain specificity for the habituating stimulus transfer, which is manifested by the presence of a modification in responses evoked either by patterns of vestibular stimulation different from those used to provoke habituation or by other sensory stimulation, such as optokinetic stimulation.

Habituation is a specific phenomenon. The possibility of obtaining unilateral habituation by unidirectional vestibular stimulations suggests that habituation is due to selective mechanisms that modify not only the gain but also the dynamic characteristics of the VOR. Unilateral habituation to step stimulation has been shown in the cat. VOR habituation is direction-specific. It proves that right and left VOR pathways can be controlled separately in order to obtain a greater system adaptability. Habituation is a central mechanism for which vestibular stimulation is not a necessary condition, since exposure to purely nonvestibular input leads to vestibular habituation. The production of nystagmus by the habituating stimulus seems unrelated to the efficacy. The habituating stimulus must produce the same subjective sensation of motion as that produced by true body motion in order to habituate vestibular nystagmus. Habituation represents the simplest type of *negative learning:* stimuli that have lost their significance for the individual are eliminated.

Compensation describes another type of central nervous counterregulation as a result of functional deterioration due to a vestibular or other equilibrium lesion. It utilizes supplementary functions which are added so that an overlay of additionally activated functions cover the underlying equilibrium lesions by means of its neuronal plasticity. However, the primary lesion continues to exist, and can, in the case of a particular conflict, manifest itself in the clinical phenomenology. Compensation is a term used in the context of phenomena which are described after unilateral failure of vestibular function. Restricted to the vestibular sphere, it includes those phenomena which cause the imbalance of vestibulo-ocular and vestibulospinal responses seen immediately after an acute unilateral failure of the vestibular system to disappear. This compensation at the vestibular level consists of the disappearance of all asymmetries (static and dynamic) in the ocular and spinal vestibular responses. In many cases substitutive interactions by visual and proprioceptive systems are required as well as some more central processes of reorganization of the reflexes in order to reach a sufficient adaptation level. Compensation is a *learning* process. The phenomenon resembles a sensorimotor relearning process implicating the activity of many integrative CNS structures. Active sensorimotor exploration provides the information to detect the errors and to correct them. Repetition of trials favors the restructure of the motor programs. Compensation implies reorganization of the remaining structures. Changes induced by the lesion as such would not necessarily lead to functionally appropriate adaptation, but rather to randomly formed synapses which may or may not be mismatched to functional needs. This "rewiring" does not result in functionally meaningless outcome, but rather leads to a new and complex circuitry, the activity of which is appropriate for the restoration of normal function. It is a goal-directed process induced by some recognized "error" in the system and directed to its elimination. Thus compensation may be defined as an error-controlled–goal-directed learning process.

These phenomena lead to different levels of recovery, which is essentially due to the integration of different levels of substitution:

– *Sensorial* substitution, in which the movement of the subject is identical to the one before the lesion but the subject uses different sets of sensory receptors for triggering and control.

– *Functional* substitution, in which the neuronal mechanisms subtending the movement have been changed but still belong to the subsystems normally used by the subject.

– *Behavioral* substitution, by which the nervous system calls for new motor behaviors not belonging to its normal repertoire.

Knowledge of the recovery phenomena following an equilibrium disturbance is fundamental for planning a correct treatment. Interpretation of recovery phenomena according to the MCS model allows correct MCS planning.

The acute vestibular lesion is a good model for explaining the main neurophysiological processes involved in the recovery of equilibrium function. Its evolution has been broadly studied in animals and it can be schematically subdivided into different stages:

– Critical stage: immediately after the lesion, the animal exhibits severe symptoms of imbalance including rapid spontaneous nystagmus, severe head deviation and forced circling and rolling toward the deafferented side.

– Acute stage: this is marked by a rapid partial recovery of asymmetry.

– Compensatory stage: the animal's recovery becomes maximal.

The duration of each period is species dependent as is also the level of recovery achieved.

From another point of view the evolution of a lesion can be interpreted as three stages of damage:

– Primary damage: the lesion that induces the onset of symptomatology

– Secondary damage: the pathological modification of the compensatory systems

– Tertiary damage: chronicization of pathologically adaptive phenomena.

Treatment must be aimed at limiting primary damage (usually by means of pharmacotherapy), to reduce secondary damage and to avoid tertiary damage.

According to the MCS model, we can simplify the course of the disease, hypothesizing that the phenomena act separately and independently from each other.

The first *mechanism* following a vestibular injury is adaptation, acting by activation of the internuclear inhibition that aims to reduce the activity of the healthy vestibular nuclei. In compensation considered at the vestibular level, the commissural fibers play an important role, especially for dynamic compensation. The influence of the remaining labyrinth upon the deafferented nucleus can take place via the commissural fibers, which are the natural means of reciprocal influence. Another early mechanism is the inhibitory influence of cerebellum, which has been called the "first-line defense" and is considered a reset to zero as a preliminary requirement for the subsequent recalibration process. This can be considered a *mechanics* phase of compensation. This phase is activated by feedback signals.

Vestibular inhibition is supported by the first compensation phenomenon: sensorial substitution. In particular, vision experience is critical for the acquisition and maintenance of recovery for the abnormally reduced VOR gain created by unilateral vestibular lesions. There has been evidence for the effect of darkness upon the evolution of the lateral head-tilt, in the cat, after hemilabyrinthectomy. When put back in the dark at a late postoperative stage, already compensated animals lose their symmetrical head position. Static visual input is a necessary condition for compensation of both ocular and postural deficits. Vision provides a sensory supply in place of the deficient vestibular supply. This supposes an increased sensitivity of the neurons of the vestibular nuclei for fast changes in the environment. Sensorial substitution is rapidly followed by and is based on the law of redundancy. The equilibrium system is a multisensorial system. In this way a vestibular sensorial input deficit may be compensated by reducing the inhibition of cervical or other proprioceptive information, or increasing visual inputs to the vestibular nuclei. The choice of which sensorial input will substitute for the lost input is based on individual preference.

The second phase is recalibration, which requires modification of the calibration of the subsystems. It is often accompanied by habituation phenomena. This can be considered the *cybernetics* phase of compensation.

The last phase of compensation is radical reorganization of the ES. The law is equifinality, that is behavioral substitution. Sensorial inputs, activity of vestibular nuclei, motor outputs and in general sensorimotor schemata are reorganized to allow the same function: equilibrium. Structural reorganization leads to a total or partial recovery of function and involves plastic structural changes and/or more global functional rearrangements of the neuronal networks, which are generally considered as the main processes underlying behavioral adaptations. This is the *synergetics* phase. This is the ultimate goal of the treatment.

According to the considerations of recovery phenomena, we can state that the therapeutic treatment must be planned according to three different levels:

1. *Mechanics:* enforcement of extensor muscles, mobilization of the main joints such as the ankle and hip. The patient acts into the environment.
2. *Cybernetics:* interaction between ocular and spinal performances. The patient interacts with the environment.
3. *Synergetics:* integration of cognitive and movement performances. The patient learns from the environment.

During the treatment, according to the MCS method, the therapist must keep in mind that the key word is *learning*. We need to teach the patient how to achieve equilibrium function and to maintain it in an unconscious way. Rehabilitation is a *teaching* process that begins in the brainstem and cerebellum and leads to a radical reorganization of both subcortical and cortical sensorimotor schema. In the following pages we will show the principle of each MCS phase of treatment and the instrument that we use for specific mechanics, cybernetics or synergetics purposes.

4.1 Mechanics Phase

Although vertigo and dizziness are caused by complex involvement of the equilibrium system, involving either primary lesions or compensatory adaptations, the mechanics phase of treatment can directly resolve the primary lesion if it is caused by musculoskeletal impairments such as weakness or a limited joint range of motion.

Musculoskeletal impairments are, more often, secondary to vestibular pathologies and they result from increased muscle tension, fatigue and pain in the cervical and, sometimes, in the thoracolumbar region. Changes in a patient's internal perception of the vertical can lead to abnormal alignment of body parts with respect to each other and to the base of support. Abnormal alignment may place patients close to their limits of stability and may alter the movement strategies necessary to move their center of gravity.

Mechanics exercises are aimed at solving musculoskeletal problems both primary and secondary, to prepare the patient's muscles, spine and joints for cybernetics and synergetics exercises, which will prepare the reorganization of the equilibrium.

Relaxation Exercises

The first step is to prepare the patient for cooperation in a complex program involving movement, thinking and learning. Musculoskeletal impairments are often provoked or associated with tension and anxiety. This is very important for starting treatment with simple relaxation exercises.

Physiotherapy

Simple exercises must be planned and they are generally aimed at mobilization of the pelvis, the cervical rachis and the thoracolumbar spine. In some cases massage can be useful either to relax the patient or to mobilize the joints.

Ski Training Oscillating Platform

The "Skitter" (Experta, Milan) is a ski training platform consisting of an oscillating plate on which two footpads are placed. Each footpad moves anteroposteriorly (toes up and toes down) and laterally, also allowing torsional movement of each foot. The plate on which the two footpads are placed "surfs" on a small oscillating table (Fig. 4.1). The oscillations of the table are slowed by several elastic cords, which regulate the resistance that the device gives to patient movements. These movements of the feet, and especially surfing and oscillating the body, simulate the movements performed during skiing (Fig. 4.2).

Some of the exercises on the Skitter were proposed either for sport training or for fitness. We have employed the Skitter for proprioceptive reeducation, especially in cases of post-traumatic unsteadiness and dizziness, because it allows the use of cognitively involved exercises and the improvement of sensorial coordination when visual feedback is associated.

For successful reeducation of reflexes by this method, cooperation of the subject is needed. The timely employment of a reeducator or of a physiotherapist offers a better chance of success.

The main *mechanics* exercises performed on the Skitter are:

A. Backward leg extension (Fig. 4.3): with one foot on the end cap and the other across the footpad, the patient keeps his weight backwards and extends the rear leg in a controlled manner; he then re-

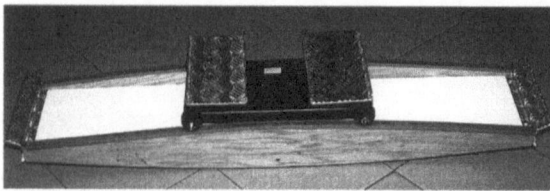

Fig. 4.1. Ski training oscillating platform: the
Skitter

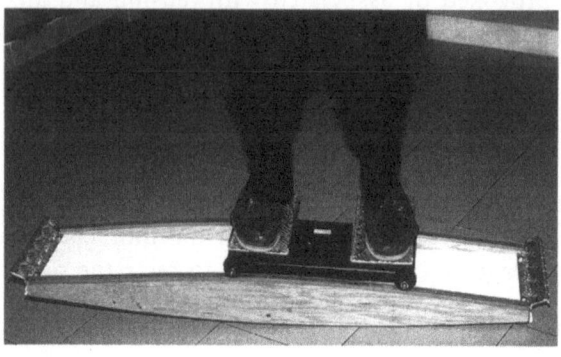

Fig. 4.2. The positions of
a skier can be reproduced
on the Skitter

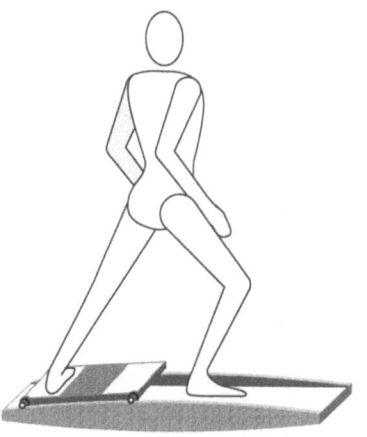

Fig. 4.3. Backward
extension

turns slowly and repeats the exercise. This improves the gluteus and
quadriceps, hamstring and trunk muscles and stabilizes the ankles
and knees.

B. Forward leg extension (Fig. 4.4)

    1. This exercise is similar to backward leg extension except the fo-
cus is on the front leg. With a stable, controlled movement, the
patient extends the leg forward to the end and repeats with both

Fig. 4.4. Forward extension

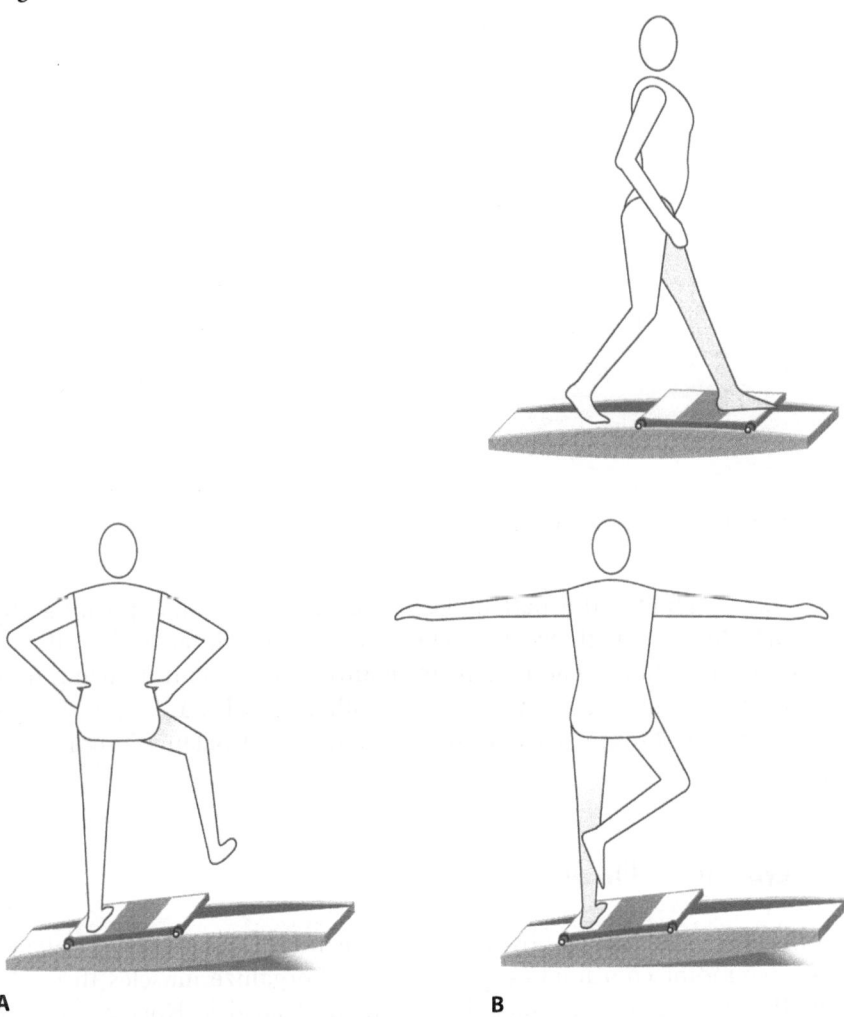

A   **B**

Fig. 4.5A, B. Standing on one leg

legs. The exercise improves the quads and trunk muscles and
stabilizes the ankles and knees.

2. The patient performs the leg extension with closed eyes to improve the self-perception of muscle tone.

C. One-leg exercise: the patient maintains equilibrium on one leg
   with the other extended (Fig. 4.5A) or flexed (Fig. 4.5B) or with
   one leg lateral. The therapist helps the patient either to maintain
   equilibrium or to correct his posture. A mirror facilitates the correction of postural equilibrium strategy.

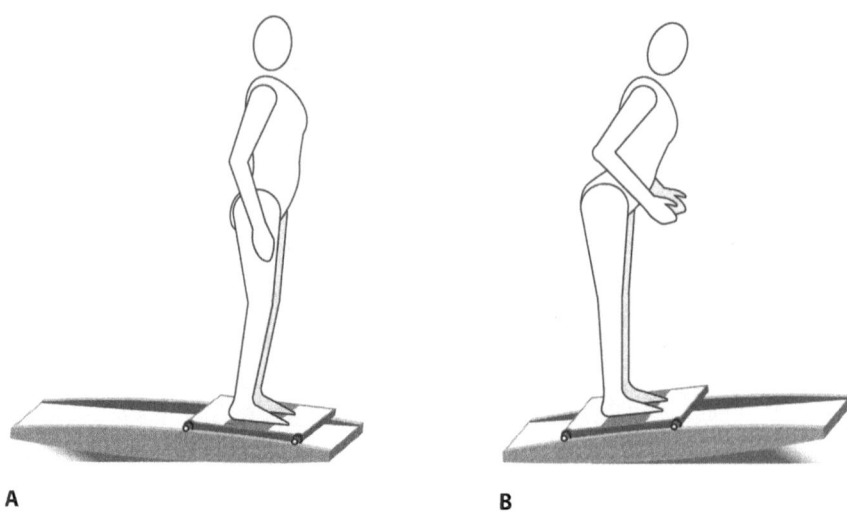

A   **B**

Fig. 4.6A, B. Exercises to improve ankle stability

D. Ankle stability: the patient keeps the knees straight pushing the skate forward with the toes (Fig. 4.6A) and pulling back with the heels (Fig. 4.6B). The patient is required to concentrate using only the ankles and calves, while all the other muscles are relaxed. This exercise improves calf and ankle stability and balance proprioception.

4.2 Cybernetics Phase

Controlling the body's position in space for the purpose of balance requires motor coordination processes that organize muscles throughout the body into coordinated movement strategies. Normal posture control requires the ability to adapt motor strategies to changing task and environmental demands. The inability to adapt movements to changing task demand is a characteristic of many patients. The pathology within the vestibular system can affect the selection of a movement strategy rather than the latency of onset or the temporal and spatial characteristics of the movement synergy itself. Patients with loss of vestibular sensitivity lose the ability to use large hip/trunk movements to control equilibrium, whereas vestibular patients with irritative lesions may use excessive hip/trunk motions for postural sway.

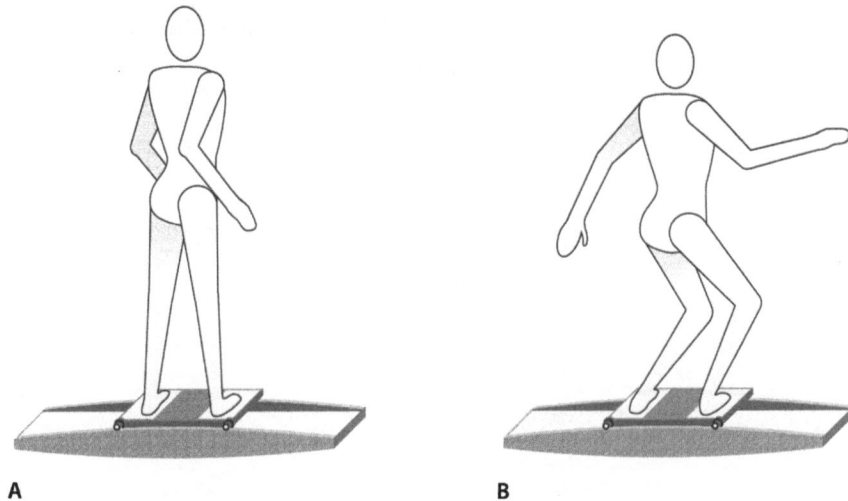

Fig. 4.7. Movements to improve ankle (**A**) and hip (**B**) strategies

Cybernetics exercises are aimed at correcting postural synergies under three different task conditions: (1) self-initiated postural sway, (2) externally induced postural responses, and (3) anticipatory postural adjustments accompanying a potentially destabilizing limb movement.

Reorganization of the equilibrium system is achieved by communicating with the environment.

Ski Training Oscillating Platform

A. Ankle-hip strategies: the patient steps on the footpads with the feet centrally positioned. He then concentrates on a proper posture using a mirror to see his reflection and transfers his weight from one foot to the other with a smooth flowing motion. During this smooth and rhythmic weight transfer the therapist induces body movements to improve ankle (Fig. 4.7A) or hip strategies (Fig. 4.7B).

B. Visual feedback: the patient stands in a comfortable and stable position on the footpads. With his thumbs and limbs extended he tries to touch visual targets placed in different positions on a facing mirror.

C. Oscillations: the patient steps on the footpads with the feet centrally positioned. Then he concentrates on a proper posture using a mirror to see his reflection. With eyes closed he transfers his

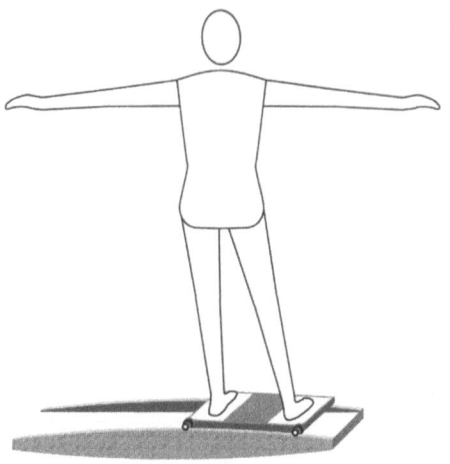

Fig. 4.8. Oscillations on the Skitter as in slalom

weight from one foot to the other with a smooth flowing motion. During this smooth and rhythmic weight transfer the therapist pushes the bumpers at one end of the Skitter, inducing a sudden and unpredictable inclination of the device.

D. Slalom (Fig. 4.8): the patient steps on the footpads with the feet centrally positioned. He then concentrates on a proper posture using a mirror to see his reflection and begins to transfer his weight from one foot to the other with a smooth flowing motion. As his rhythms increase he moves closer to the bumpers at each end, always maintaining a good upright posture with eyes focused in the mirror and paying attention to his balance. If the exercise is performed with limited upper body movement (such as in slalom), it improves the hip rotators, quadriceps and calves while it also stimulates the abdominal stabilizers and gluteus muscles when the patient includes upper body motion (such as in giant slalom). The exercises are performed concentrating on the proper edge-setting techniques.

Vestibular Electrical Stimulation

Electrical stimulation (ES) is a noninvasive technique that provides nerve and/or muscle stimulation by means of surface electrodes. The characteristics, size and site of application of the electrodes and the characteristics of the electrical waves play a fundamental role in the neurophysiological effects of the ES. Usually hand-held antalgic electrostimulators are called TENS (transcutaneous electrical nerve stimu-

Fig. 4.9. The device used for vestibular electrical stimulation

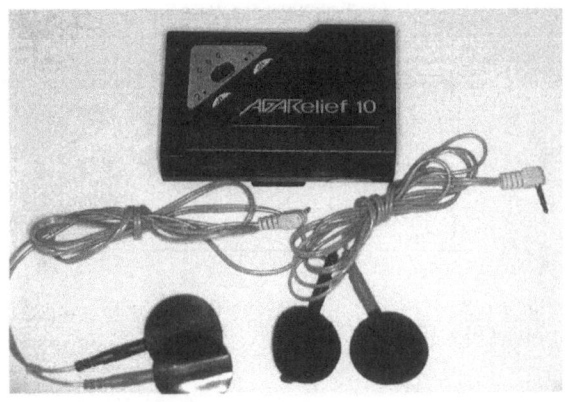

lation) stimulators. This definition can be considered deceiving. The excitation of the peripheral motor nerves and the associated muscle activation is caused by the application of an electric current to the skin, usually corresponding to the motor points. This kind of stimulation induces depolarization of the motor nerves either in a centrifugal or in a centripetal direction. Furthermore this kind of stimulation induces an activation of the sensitive nerves of the skin. Thus it is difficult to distinguish the motor and the sensitive effects of the ES.

As is known, vibration is the specific exogenous stimulation of proprioceptors of the paravertebral muscles. Our previous experimental experience has shown that vibration of the paravertebral muscles can be substituted for with electrical stimulation. Lackner (1993) remarked that the vestibular nuclei are really multisensorial relays and that they are not only related to labyrinth activity. The author underlined that it is not possible under natural circumstances to activate the vestibular receptors without implicating other force-sensitive receptor systems that convey information relevant to spatial orientation.

On the basis of this extensive, but physiologically justified, point of view of the vestibular system, we named the superficial paravertebral electrical stimulation *vestibular electrostimulation* (VES).

For both experimentation and clinical application we use an Agar electrostimulator, which is a small (25×36×91 mm) and light (88 g) portable device manufactured at Hadassah University Hospital, Jerusalem (Israel), and approved by the USA Food and Drug Administration (Fig. 4.9). The mean currency intensity is 0.9 $\mu A/mm^2$, the impulse currency intensity is 30 $\mu A/mm^2$, the maximum impulse power is 5 W, the maximum impulse charge is 22 μC and the mean impulse charge is 0.55 C.

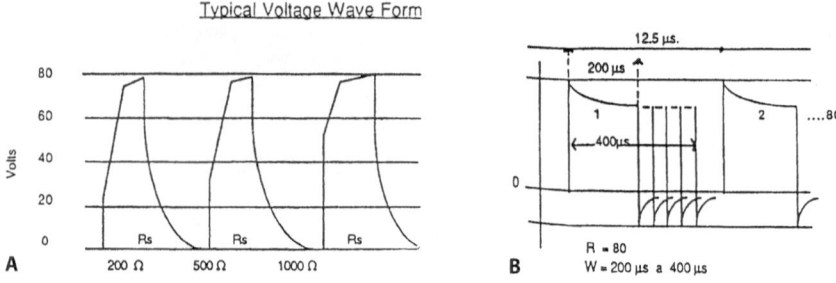

Fig. 4.10A, B. The typical wave that provides the stimulation able to induce vestibular-like effects

The device is able to produce different stimulation modes such as the "burst," which consists of a short pulse series at a high frequency repeated at slow frequency. This stimulation mode is used for pain relief. The stimulation should be strong enough that muscle contractions can be seen. Usually the electrode is placed on a large muscle near to the aching spot. The "burst" is not useful for vestibular stimulation, although it can sometimes be used for mechanics enforcement of the muscles of the legs.

VES consists of a biphasic asymmetrical modulated square wave (Fig. 4.10). The modulation program randomly modifies the duration of each wave. The mean duration is 100 µs while the frequency is 80 Hz. The electrodes are small (2 cm^2) placed a distance of 1 cm from each other. A pair of electrodes stimulates the paravertebral muscles at the level of the second cervical vertebra, one pair stimulating the contralateral superior trapezius. The intensity of VES is never able to induce muscle contractions. The frequency used is in the muscle spindle range of vibratory activation (80 Hz). Thus, it is likely that VES activates the same spinal pathways as the cervicospinal reflexes. It modulates the lower limb postural reflexes in the same way.

Vibratory stimulation of muscle stimulation in a range between 1 and 100 Hz is able to activate muscle spindles. The vibratory stimulation of the neck muscles produces proprioceptive inputs to the brainstem. These afferent volleys are able to evoke postural reflexes from the muscle of the lower limbs, cervicospinal reflexes, by means of the same mechanism. Vibration is also able to evoke alterations of the perceptual representation of the shape and orientation of the whole body and/or body parts.

The experimental results obtained by means of VES show that this kind of stimulation clearly influences the excitability of the motor neurons of the lower limbs. This influence resembles the action of cervicospinal reflexes on the extensor lower muscles.

Alteration of proprioceptive input from the neck by VES leads to a changed perception of head position and the manipulated proprioceptive input is incorporated in the head position signal with other inputs contributing to head and body position control.

Exercises with the Soft Mattress: The Rettiks

The "Rettiks" (Experta, Milan) is a foam mattress that destabilizes the ankles and reduces the information from the feet. To maintain equilibrium the patient must make the best possible use of visual and vestibular information. It consists of three segments with a total length of 3 m. The external parts slope gradually from a height of 1 cm to 10 cm. The central segment is 10 cm high. The material differs from the usual foam mattress. It has a certain plasticity and, when it is deformed, it returns the applied forces slowly, making it difficult for the patient to adapt. The sensation that the patient feels when walking on it is like that in snow or on sand and the foot is unable to find a stable surface for support. The conformation of the mattress allows different exercises, either standing or walking. In the standing position the height of the foam can be graduated from a few centimeters up to 30 cm by overlapping two or three segments and by placing the patient at one extremity or in the center of the inclined segments (Fig. 4.11).

Standing Exercises (Fig. 4.12)

A. The patient stands in front of a mirror with his legs apart. He tries to maintain equilibrium (Fig. 4.13 A) also using the arms (Fig. 4.13 B).
B. In the same position the therapist destabilizes the patient (Fig. 4.13 C–D).
C. The patient moves the body with or without the arms with a narrow support base or
D. Crossing his legs.

Walking Exercises

A. The three segments are aligned. The patient walks slowly over the mattress first with the eyes open then with the eyes closed (Fig. 4.14).

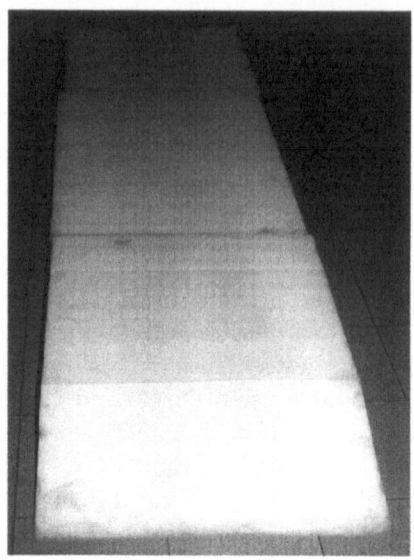

Fig. 4.11. The Rettiks soft mattress

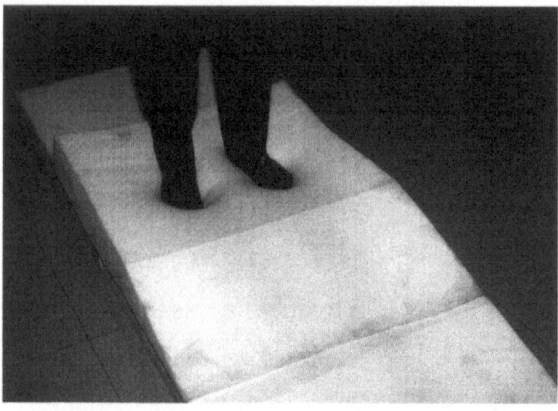

Fig. 4.12. Equilibrium on the soft mattress with and without destabilization

B. The segments are partially overlapped. The path is characterized by steps. The patient walks first with the eyes open, then closed, and finally moving his head.

C. Stepping on one (Fig. 4.15 A) or two overlapped segments (Fig. 4.15 B).

It is also possible to perform different exercises lying on the mattress. The most effective are those require arm-leg synchronization such as in the quadrupedal position (Fig. 4.16).

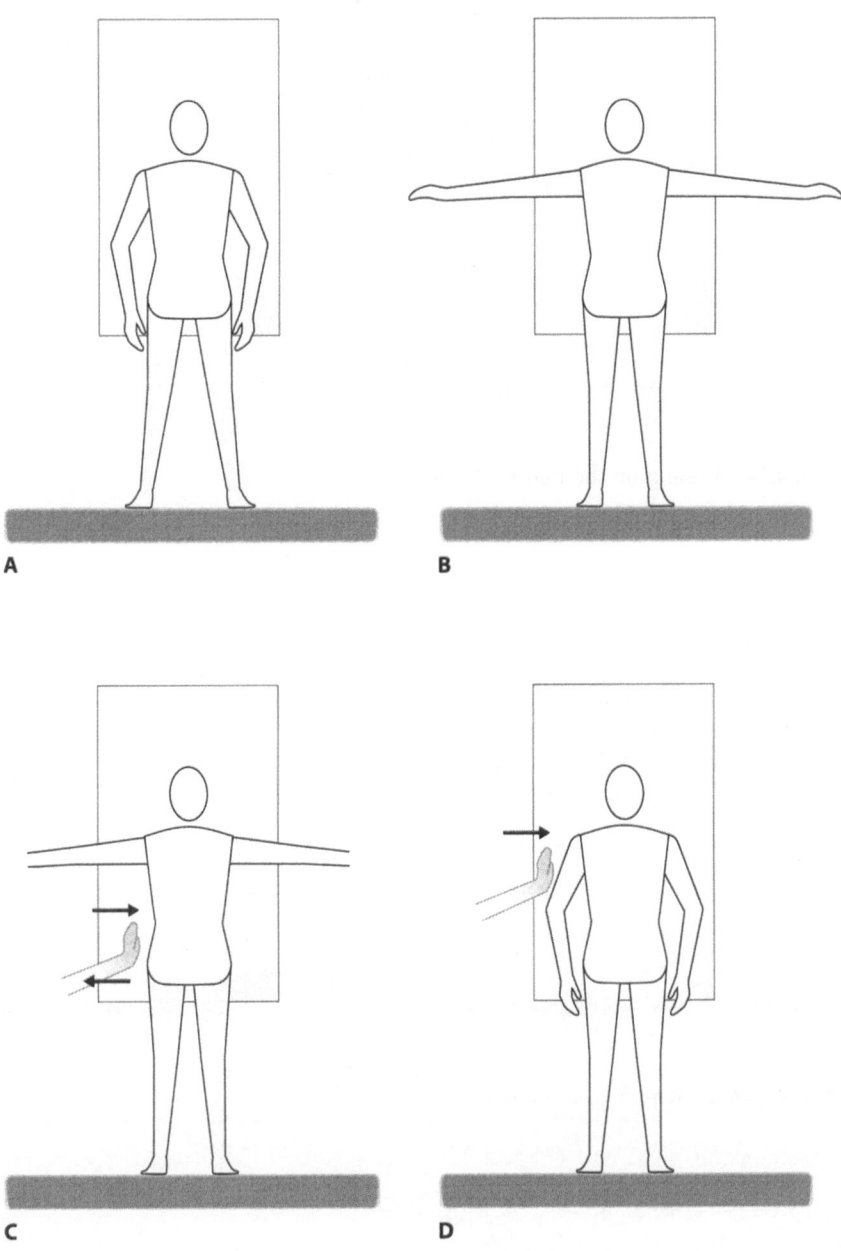

Fig. 4.13 A–D. Standing exercises

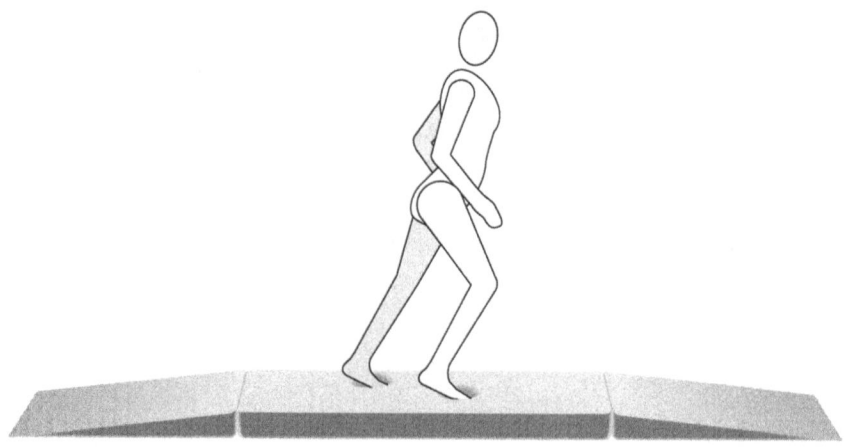

Fig. 4.14. Walking on the Rettiks "path"

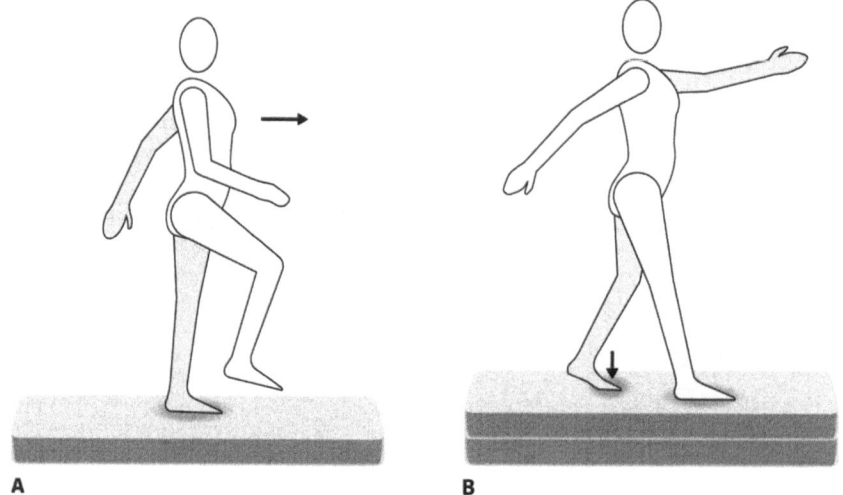

A

B

Fig. 4.15 A, B. Stepping on the Rettiks

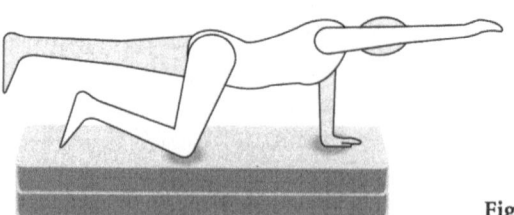

Fig. 4.16. Arm-leg synchronization

Visual Prisms

Prisms have been employed in the treatment of vertigo since the 1940s, when Unthermohlen (1941) described their utilization in the treatment of Meniere's disease. Then Baron used them in patients after head trauma, with scoliosis and with paralysis of extrinsic ocular muscles. Prisms divert light onto the retina and they cause an apparent displacement of an object. In this way the eyes modify their position in the orbit to maintain fixation. This activates the proprioceptive chain, modifying the activity of the extensor muscles with special regards to those of the legs. Prisms in MCS rehabilitation are used in three situations:

A. To displace the eyes in a non-nystagmic position when oscillopsia due to spontaneous nystagmus is present (such as in acute unilateral vestibular hypofunction). They are placed with their bases on the side of the spontaneous nystagmus direction (the eyes displaces to the opposite side).

B. To activate the proprioceptive chain. For example, to activate right extensory oculopostural reactions, prisms are placed with the bases on the left.

C. To enhance VOR by means of vergence activation. In this case both bases are placed toward the outer direction of gaze.

Prisms are then used to correct convergence deficits in patients affected with structural fragility syndrome.

4.3 Synergetics Phase

Balance deficits can result from damage within individual sensory systems which provide spatial orientation information, or from pathology affecting central sensory structures important in the interpretation and selection of sensory information for balance control. Disruption of the synergetics phase of equilibrium control may affect coordination and orientation perception (that is to say causing vertigo and dizziness) in several ways: (1) a patient's ability to accurately determine the orientation of the body with respect to gravity and the environment may be disturbed, (2) a patient's ability to adapt sensory inputs to changes in task and environmental demand may be impaired and (3) a patient's ability to anticipate instability based on prior experience may be affected.

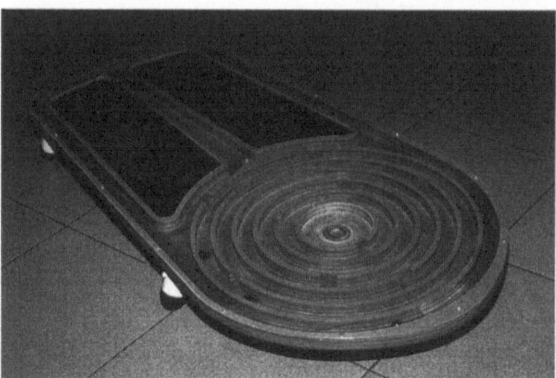

Fig. 4.17. Labyrinth on an undulating platform: the Daedalus

Synergetics exercises are aimed at reducing uncoordination and disorientation and their consciousness, through *learning from* the environment new movement strategies and correct orientation.

Rettiks

A. The patient stands on the mattress while reading a book. His arms are extended and he begins moving the book to and fro while reading.
B. The same exercises with the book are performed while walking over the mattress in a gradual or in a stepped path.

Daedalus: Labyrinth on an Undulating Platform

The "Daedalus" (FLEM, Treviso, Italy) is a wooden table lying on a ball. It undulates according to the position of the ball, which is not fixed, and the state of inflation of the ball. At the top of the table is a 50-cm-diameter labyrinth. A ball can be maneuvered into the labyrinth by moving the platform. Two sticks can be placed anteriorly or posteriorly in order to help the patient induce different positions of the body (Fig. 4.17). The patient stands on the platform and he can perform different exercises.

A. He maintains equilibrium with the sticks (Fig. 4.18) or without them (Fig. 4.19).
B. He tries to move the ball, running it through the labyrinth from the external circle to the center (Fig. 4.20).
C. He moves the platform while in the prone position, using the arms (Fig. 4.21).

Fig. 4.18. Moving the ball through the labyrinth also using sticks

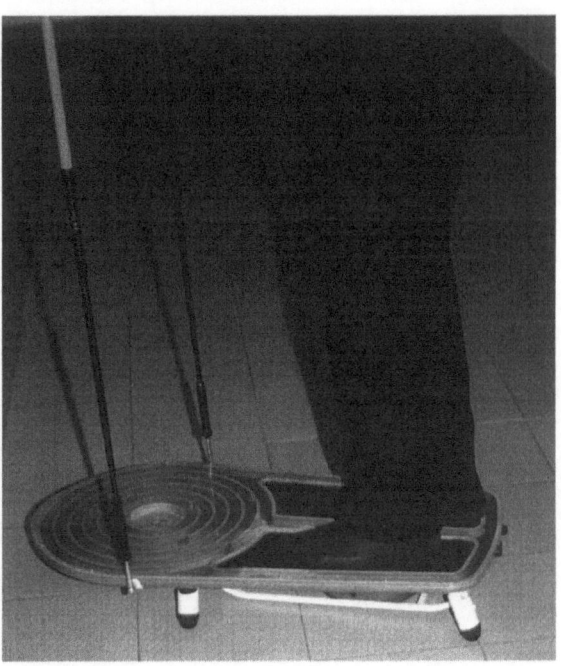

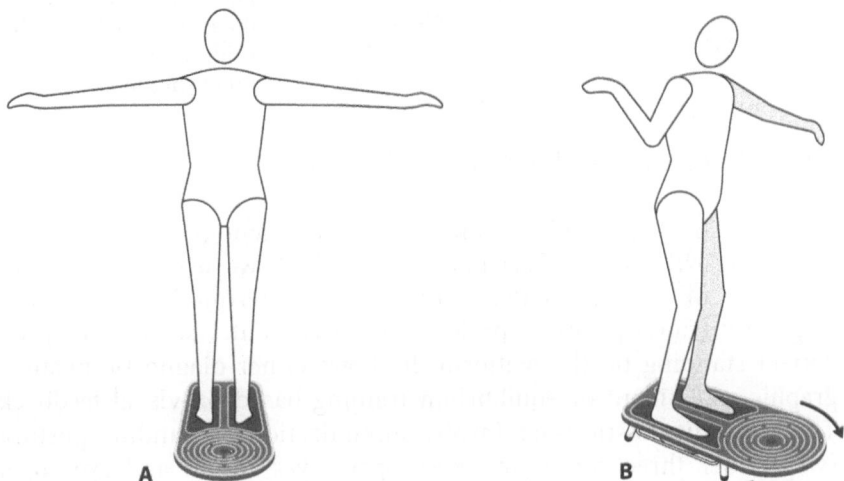

Fig. 4.19A, B. Equilibrium on the platform, without sticks

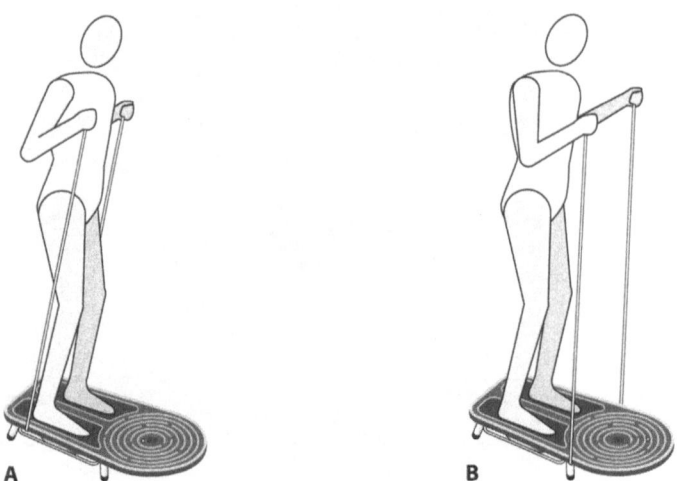

Fig. 4.20A, B. Maneuvering the ball through the labyrinth using the sticks in different positions

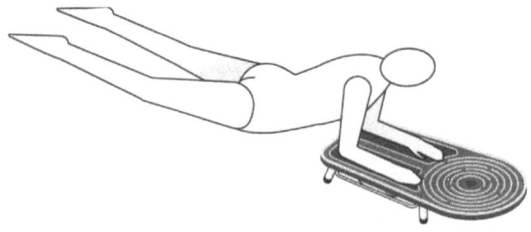

Fig. 4.21. Maneuvering the ball through the labyrinth in the prone position using the arms

Visual Feedback Stabilometric Reeducation

This stabilometric method consists of equipment (such the Balance Master by Neurocom, Clackamas, USA, which we use) that provides by means of a single or dual footplate visual feedback on the center of gravity (CoG) position, projected on a computer screen facing the patient standing on the platform. It allows either diagnostic posturographic assessment or equilibrium training based on visual feedback. The static diagnostic tasks involve minimization of standing postural sway under three conditions: eyes open, eyes closed and eyes open with visual feedback. During rehabilitative training, the patient has to move his CoG projection actively according to specific instructions regarding amplitude and velocity, received through the screen. It has been stated that if the patient becomes able to control actively his CoG movements in the standing position he will be able to transfer this skill to daily activities, in an automatic and unconscious manner.

Stabilometry presents the therapist and patient with a comprehensive program of balance rehabilitation. It provides the opportunity for both quantitative assessment and training.

The Balance Master

The Balance Master footplate consists of two 9-in. (23 cm) footplates. There is a pin joint between the two plates, 9 in. from the rear border of the plates. The axis along the pin joint constitutes the x (lateral)-axis. The pin joint also intersects the y (anteroposterior)-axis.

Each footplate rests on two force transducers with the sensitive axes oriented vertically. The transducers are mounted along the front-to-back center line of each plate (one 8.25 in. behind and the other 8.125 in. in front of the pin joint). The lateral distance between left and right plate transducers and center is 5.00 in.

The sum of the vertical forces exerted on the left footplate transducers is equal to the sum of forces on the right footplate transducers when the vertical force center is located at any point along the boundary between the two plates. This places the x-axis zero position at the y-axis.

For each footplate, the vertical forces exerted on the front and the back transducers are equal when the vertical forces exerted on the plate are centered between the front and back transducers (i.e., at the pin joint). This places the y-axis zero position at the pin joint.

The total vertical force exerted on the two footplates is calculated by summing the four vertical force signals. Anteroposterior CoG sway angle is the angle between a vertical line projecting upward from the center of the area of feet support and a second line projecting from the same point to the subject's CoG. When normal subjects maintain a vertically erect position, the CoG is located directly over the area of feet support, slightly forward of the ankle joints. This position can be maintained without stepping or reaching for support if sway does not exceed the subject's limits of stability.

Principles of Operation of Visual Feedback Stabilometry

In theory, the forward limit of stability places the CoG over the front boundary of the support area; the backward stability limit places the CoG over the back boundary of the support area. In practice, the effective limits of stability are somewhat smaller than would be predicted by foot length, since in most individuals the strength of the intrinsic foot muscles prevents the full body weight being borne by the toes or the extreme backs of the heels.

Functional stability limits have been calculated to be 6.25° anteriorly and 4.45° posteriorly for the average adult subject. The angular limits of stability are very nearly the same for all adults regardless of height.

When a subject is standing quietly on the forceplate with ankles placed symmetrically over the electrical center of forceplate, the vertical projection of CoG is assumed to intersect the forceplate at the center of vertical force position. As the body moves more rapidly, the vertical projection of the CoG lags increasingly behind the center of vertical force.

When CoG sway is a reflection of the body rotating as a rigid mass about the ankle joints, there are no horizontal components of force exerted against the support surface. In contrast, hip movement generates horizontal forces against the support surface that are proportional to the acceleration of the hip joint angle. Changes in vertical force position during hip movement only occur when the hip movement also causes changes in the CoG sway angle.

To maintain stability with the feet in place, the body's center of gravity must be positioned vertically over the base of support. When this condition is met, a person can both resist the destabilizing influence of gravity and actively move the CoG. If the CoG is positioned outside the perimeter of the base of support, the person has exceeded the in-place limits of stability. At this point, to prevent falling, a rapid step or stumble to reestablish the base of support beneath the CoG or additional external support is required.

The base of support for standing on a flat, firm surface is defined as the area contained within the perimeter of contact between the surface and the two feet. The base of support area is nearly square when the feet are placed comfortably apart during quiet standing.

The limits of stability (LoS) measure is a two-dimensional quantity defining the largest possible CoG sway angle as a function of sway direction from the center position. The LoS depends on the placement of the feet and the base of support. In normal adults standing on a flat, firm surface with feet comfortably apart, the LoS perimeter can best be described as an ellipse. The AP dimension of this ellipse is approximately 12.5° from the most backward point to the most forward point on the perimeter. Although the height of the CoG above the surface and the foot length affect the AP limits of stability, these two features covary, resulting in approximately the same AP limits for persons of various heights. The lateral LoS depends on the person's height relative to the spacing between the feet. When the feet of a person 180 cm tall are placed 10 cm apart, for example, the lateral dimension of the LoS ellipse is approximately 16° from the farthest point on the left to the farthest point on the right on the perimeter.

The biomechanical properties that determine the LoS are similar for standing in place, walking and sitting without trunk support. During in-place standing the CoG moves randomly within an LoS perimeter determined by the base of support and the placement of the feet. During walking the CoG progresses forward through the LoS in a smooth rhythmic movement. At heel strike the LoS are established with the CoG positioned at the posterior perimeter. As the step progresses, the CoG moves forward within the LoS. As the CoG approaches the anterior perimeter of the LoS, the next step establishes a new LoS and the rhythmic processes are repeated. When a person is sitting without trunk support, the height of the CoG above the support surface is lower and the base area is larger. Therefore the LoS perimeter is larger when a person is seated than during quiet standing.

For these reasons reeducation of the limits of stability in standing in place can be used to rehabilitate the patient and to regain normal LoS during walking, too.

When a person's postural stability is disrupted by an external stimulus, one or a combination of three different strategies is typically used to coordinate movement of the CoG back to a balanced position. When body displacement is beyond the LoS perimeter, a step or stumbling reaction is the only movement strategy effective in preventing fall. When the CoG remains within the LoS, two different strategies or a combination thereof can be used to move the CoG while maintaining the initial placement of the feet on the support surface: the ankle strategy and the hip strategy. The correct execution of the LoS test normally requires combined and integrated ankle-hip strategies. The relative effectiveness of these two kinds of postural strategy in positioning and maintaining the CoG in the desired position (Fig. 4.22) depends on the configuration of the base support, the CoG alignment in relation to the LoS, and the speed of the postural movement.

A normal individual moves primarily about the ankles when sway amplitude is well within the LoS and increases the use of hip movement when sway approaches the LoS. Postural movements are ineffective in the patient who uses ankle strategy movements to control sway displacements of large amplitude. The patient who depends on

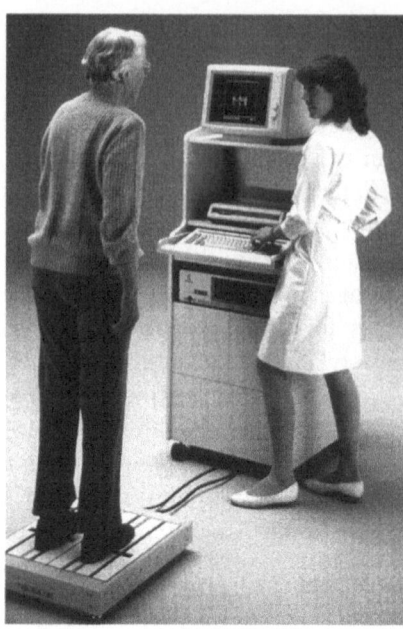

Fig. 4.22. Visual feedback stabilometry: the Balance Master (Balance Master, reproduced by courtesy of NeuroCom International, Inc., Clackamas, Oregon, USA)

ankle movements falls prematurely when sway amplitude is large. The patient using hip movements to control sway of small amplitude is inefficient and expends a needlessly high level of energy to maintain a centered CoG position. Ineffective use of movement strategies may be caused by abnormal adaptation or by an inability to produce one of the two movement patterns, for example, inappropriate use of the hip movement during sway of small amplitude caused by anxiety or by misperception of the LoS. Anxiety and LoS misperception are common findings in whiplash patients. In these cases training aimed at teaching the appropriate conditions for using ankle movements can have a positive impact. In contrast, weakness of ankle joint muscles, loss of ankle sensation, reduced mobility about the ankles, or combinations of these factors prevent the patient from generating effective ankle movements and might be an abnormal adaptation used by the dizzy patient to minimize head movements and associated stimulation of the neck and the vestibular system. Distortion of the somatosensory inputs from the ankles alters the displacement of the head whether the eyes are open or closed, and visual information is necessary to coordinate specific postural patterns utilizing horizontal shear forces to maintain a stance on a mechanically compliant surface. The control of the head position during balance is also dependent on somatosensory inputs from the feet or lower limbs which are generated by foot contact with the supporting surface.

Shumway-Cook et al. (1991) conducted the first study that used objective visual feedback, based on symmetry of postural sway (movement of the CoG), for training purposes. This study compared the effectiveness of visual feedback with more conventional physical therapy techniques for reestablishing symmetry of standing in hemiparetic patients. During sessions, the therapist also gave tactile and verbal cues to assist patients in maintaining good postural alignment.

Regarding Balance Master training, the duration of each treatment session is 20 min. The frequency of treatment generally varies from twice a week to every day. The frequency of training sessions is dependent on a combination of other rehabilitative treatments such as physical therapy and vestibular electrical stimulation.

Visual feedback provides information about postural instability for both the patient and the therapist. The purpose of visual feedback is to detect and make available to the patient objective information about physiological function or movement that is not ordinarily perceived by the patient. In the case of postural instability, visual, and auditory (beep), signals have been used to give the patient information about head and trunk orientation and about symmetry of weight bearing through the lower extremities. The assumption is that the patient can use visual or auditory cues better than he or she could use somatosensation or vestibular inputs.

For the therapist stabilometry establishes a baseline of patient function, facilitates the design of custom treatments (Fig. 4.23) and evaluates the effectiveness of the therapeutic program. For the patient it

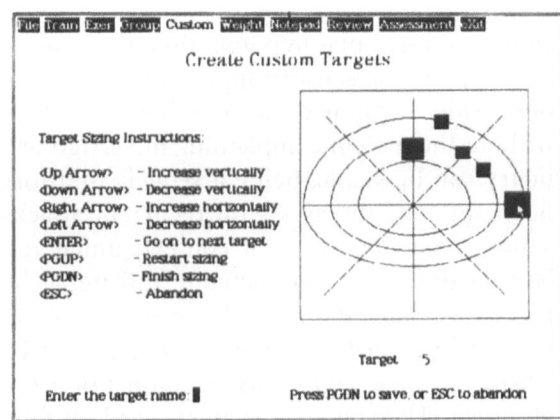

Fig. 4.23. Preparation of feedback program (Balance Master, reproduced by courtesy of NeuroCom International, Inc., Clackamas, Oregon, USA)

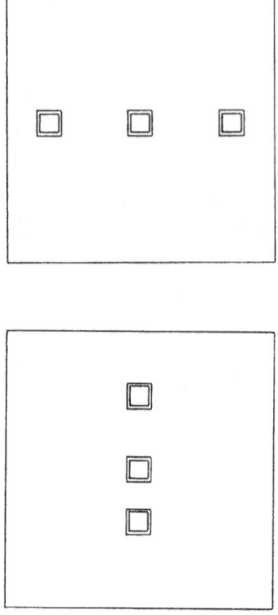

Fig. 4.24. An example of the target position to improve laterolateral movements (Balance Master, reproduced by courtesy of NeuroCom International, Inc., Clackamas, Oregon, USA)

Fig. 4.25. An example of the target position to improve anteroposterior strategies (Balance Master, reproduced by courtesy of NeuroCom International, Inc., Clackamas, Oregon, USA)

enhances motivation through real-time visual feedback, links perception to movement, internalizes the appropriate alignment or movement pattern, improves volitional control and builds confidence to perform the activities of daily living (Figs. 4.24, 4.25).

4.4 MCS Protocols

Acute Unilateral Vestibular Hypofunction

Unilateral vestibular hypofunction means asymmetrical vestibular functioning, i.e., the sensory input of one side is diminished relative to the other side. Asymmetrical peripheral functioning can also be detected without the patient complaining of vertigo or instability. Such an asymmetry can be stable, being a sequela of a former lesion. It can also be fluctuant, e.g., in cases with recurrent attacks of Meniere's disease. In a more restricted clinical context, unilateral vestibular hypofunction is considered as nonfluctuant unilateral loss, where compensation plays a fundamental role. The most striking form is the syndrome with sudden loss. In this syndrome (described by Stenger and Frenzel in 1965), the same signs and symptoms of a postlabyrinthectomy can be observed. The course is characterized by four stages:

1. Stage of irritation: in some cases the onset of the syndrome may be characterized by a rather vague dizziness. At this moment the spontaneous nystagmus beats towards the affected side and normal caloric reaction can be observed.
2. Stage of sudden loss of function, or paralysis of the system; typical rotatory vertigo is now experienced and spontaneous nystagmus beats towards the normal side. The caloric reaction is absent or reduced on the affected side. Patients generally visit the emergency room of the hospital during this stage, and hospitalization is common.
3. Stage of central compensation: there is a progressive decrease of vertigo as well as of spontaneous nystagmus. This occurs independently of the persistence of unilateral weakness or areflexia on the affected side revealed by caloric stimulations. Provocative maneuvers (especially head shaking) reveal vertigo and nystagmus.
4. Stage of recovery: when the function of the affected side recovers, this may lead to a spontaneous nystagmus, reversed in direction, i.e., beating towards the affected side.

The following protocol is for the rehabilitative treatment of patients during the stage of sudden loss of vestibular function.

Hospital Treatment

In the early phase of acute vertigo, symptoms are characterized by nausea and vomiting; and rotatory vertigo is present in every position of the head and the body with a slight decrease in symptoms on the opposite site of the lesion, oscillopsia due to nystagmus, and unsteadiness with typical standing and gait deviations toward the affected side. The first mechanism of recovery is internuclear inhibition, which can lead to a bilateral reduction of the vestibular responses. The cybernetics phase of recovery is featured by sensory substitution phenomena. MCS treatment aims to:
1. Reduce antigravitational failure of the affected side.
2. Reduce oscillopsia due to nystagmus.
3. Activate sensory substitution phenomena.
4. Reduce internuclear inhibition.
5. Reactivate coordination.
6. Reduce spatial disorientation (vertigo).

In the acute phase drugs are often necessary especially those that reduce neurovegetative symptoms, such as methoclopramide, and those that can potentially activate neurochemical compensation pathways such as benzodiazepine and amantadine.

The first step of the rehabilitative treatment of acute vertigo is:

Vestibular Electrical Stimulation

According to the neurophysiological evidence, electrodes must be placed on the paravertebral muscles opposite the affected site (the side of the direction of the spontaneous nystagmus) and on the trapezius of the affected side. Two stimulations a day must be performed for at least 1 h each. During the first half an hour the patient remains in bed, if possible in the most comfortable position lying on the healthy side, in the light, trying to keep the eyes open and fixating a target on the opposite side of the visual field (on the side of the affected labyrinth).

In this phase it is better if visual prisms are also used. Generally low prisms are used, e.g., 3–5°, based on the opposite side of the lesion. After half an hour of VES, the patient, under the effect of drugs, must achieve an upright position and then, accompanied by the therapist, begins walking. A walking gait must be performed during VES, wearing visual prisms, while the therapist teaches the patient to fixate a target in front of him. After some steps the patient starts his return, turning around himself. The sense of rotation must not be casual but it must be according to the side of the healthy labyrinth. Instructions for re-fixating a target must be given.

After the 1st day of treatment simple in bed exercises must be performed, twice a day, for at least 20–30 min each session:

1. The patient fixates a target on the ceiling and slowly moves his head rightward and leftward.
2. The patient looks for two equidistant targets on the ceiling and then he fixates them alternately first moving only the eyes and then moving only the head.
3. The patient rotates his head in the direction of the affected labyrinth and fixates a target on the lateral wall. He then straightens his head maintaining the visual fixation. He counts up to 10 and then he rotates his head again.
4. The patient lifts his leg on the affected side with the knee extended (Fig. 4.26).
5. He repeats this move with the tip of the foot outward.
6. He repeats the move again with the tip of the foot inward.
7. The patient puts a pillow under his leg on the affected side, a 2-kg weight is bound to his ankle with the flexed knee; then he extends it (Fig. 4.27).

Fig. 4.26. Extension of
the left knee in a case of
a lesion on the left

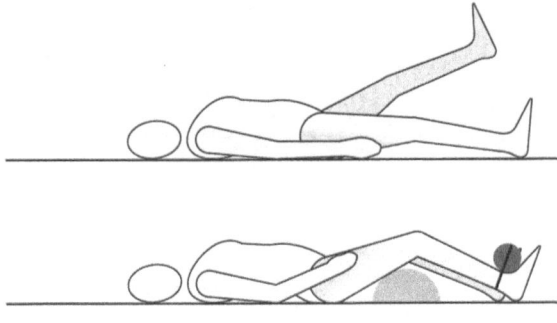

Fig. 4.27. Extension of
the right knee, binding a
weight to the ankle, in a
case of a lesion on the
right

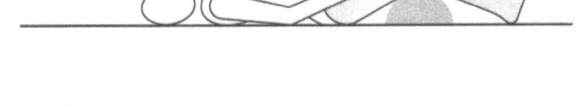

When it is possible to maintain a sitting position, the following exercises must be performed during VES and wearing visual prisms:

1. The patient extends his arms and lifts his thumbs. He moves his arms about 50 cm from his eyes, along a horizontal plane, and then he fixates each thumb alternately. He begins slowly and then increases progressively the velocity of alternate fixation.
2. The patient extends his arms and lifts his thumbs. He moves his arms at about 50 cm from his eyes, along a vertical plane, and then he fixates each thumb alternately. He begins slowly and then increases, progressively, the velocity of alternate fixation.
3. The patient extends his right arm and lifts his thumb. He moves his arm to and fro slowly, first in a horizontal direction, then in a vertical direction. He follows his thumb with the eyes only, first slowly and then increasing progressively the velocity of thumb displacement.
4. As above but simultaneously also moving the head while trying to maintain the eyes still.
5. The patient moves his head first slowly and then faster in all directions, fixating a target straight in front of him (Fig. 4.28).
6. The patient looks for three targets placed, respectively, in front of him, on his left and on his right. He fixates the frontal target, then he moves his head rapidly fixating the target on the right. He then turns his head leftward maintaining the fixation of the target on the right. He fixates the frontal target. He moves his

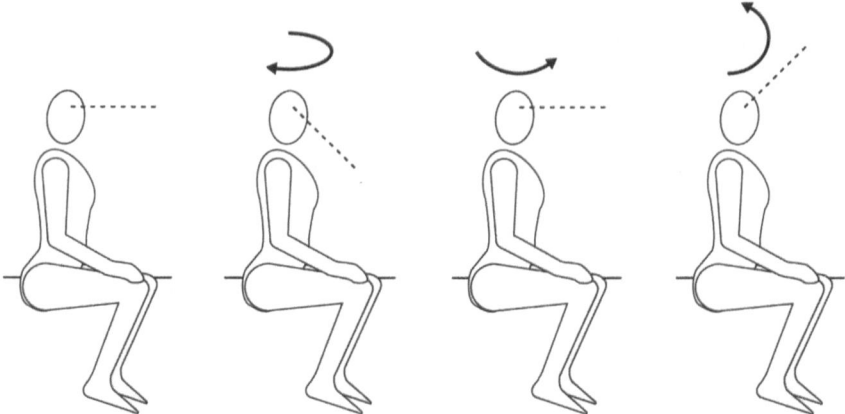

Fig. 4.28. Movements of the head in all directions fixating a target straight in front of the patient

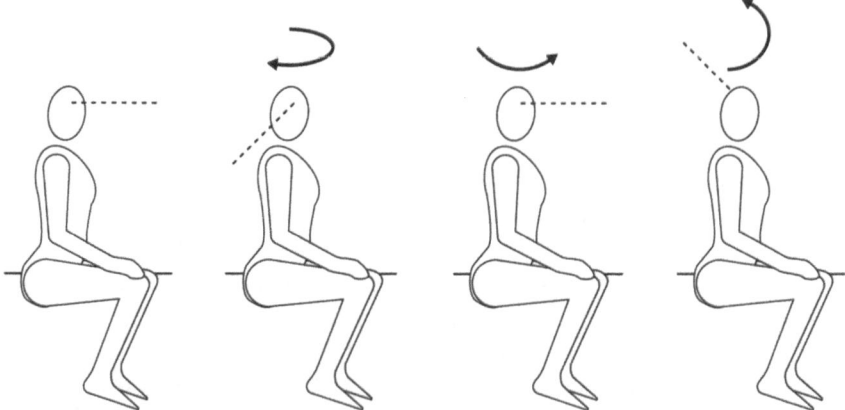

Fig. 4.29. Alternating fixation of three targets

head rapidly leftward and fixates the target on the left. He then turns his head rightward maintaining the fixation of the target on the left (Fig. 4.29).

7. The patient assumes a sitting position and fixates a target in front of him. He then lies down on the floor fixating a target on the ceiling. Then he gets up re-fixating the target in front of him (Fig. 4.30).

8. The patient sits on the bed. The therapist pushes him in order to stimulate coordinated equilibrium reaction of the body (Fig. 4.31).

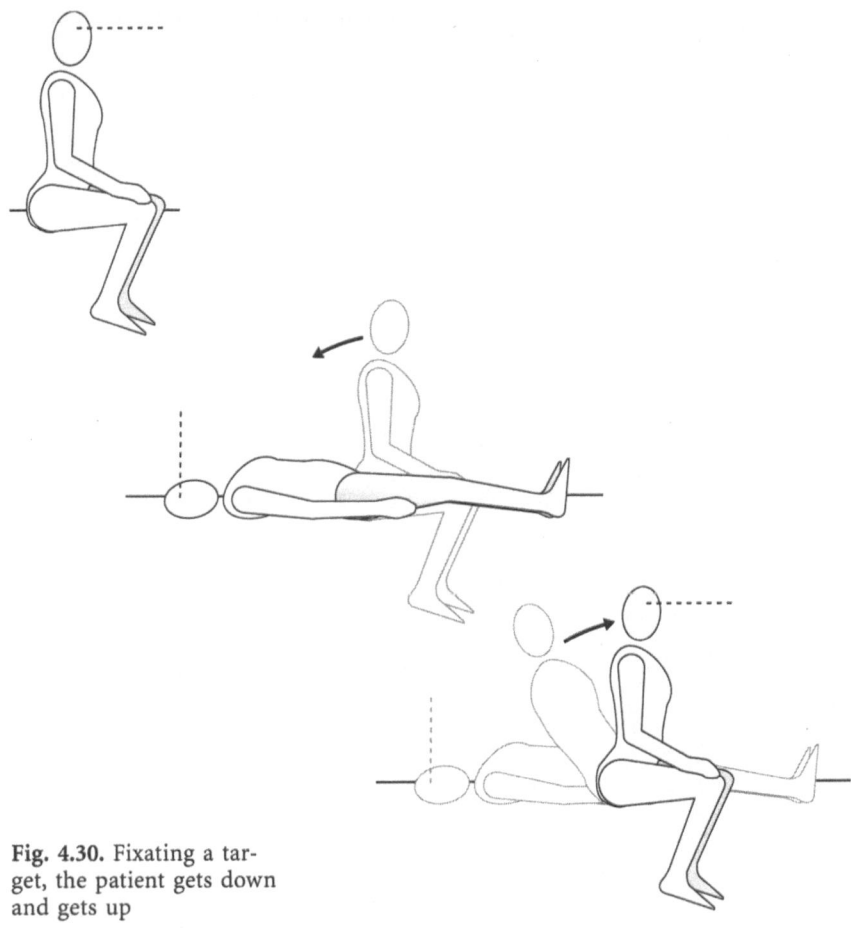

Fig. 4.30. Fixating a target, the patient gets down and gets up

9. The patient stands and the therapist stands behind the patient. The therapist pulls the patient to stimulate equilibrium reactions (Fig. 4.32).
10. As above but the therapist is in front of the patient (Fig. 4.33).
11. The patient sits on the bed and the therapist pulls him to stimulate equilibrium reactions (Fig. 4.34).
12. The patient lies supine on an oscillating table. The therapist moves the table to stimulate equilibrium reactions (Fig. 4.35).
13. The patient sits on a chair and tries to destabilize himself by standing on two legs on the same side as the affected labyrinth, while maintaining equilibrium (Fig. 4.36).

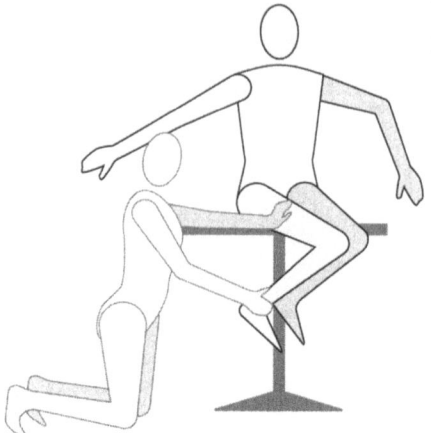

Figs. 4.31–4.35. Equilibrium reactions to pushing stimulation by the therapist

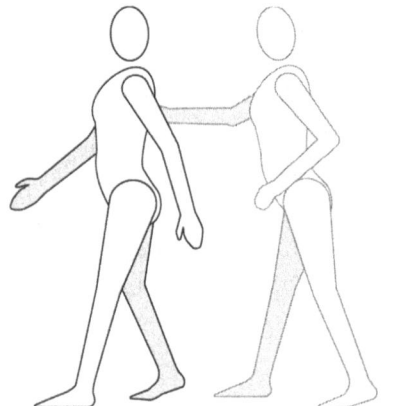

Fig. 4.32

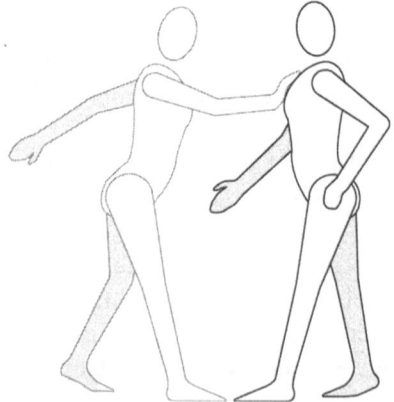

Fig. 4.33

Fig. 4.34

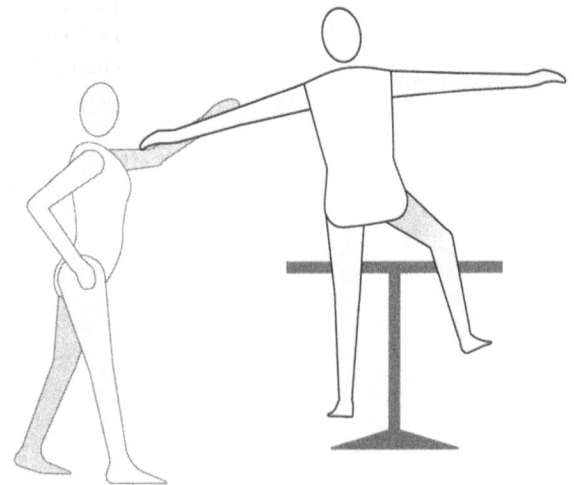

Fig. 4.35

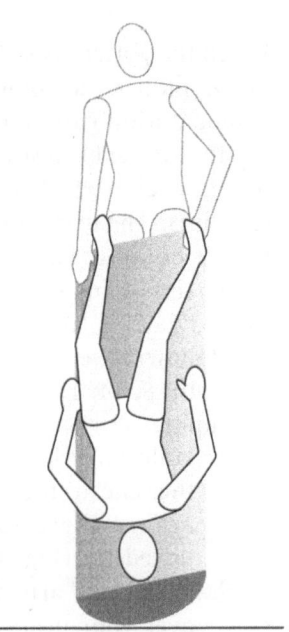

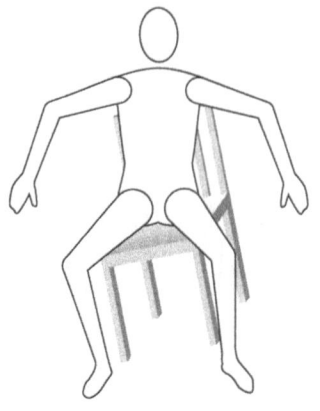

Fig. 4.36. Patient tries to maintain equilibrium in a destabilized position of the chair

Home Protocol

When the patient is sufficiently well to be able to walk alone and there is no oscillopsia, a home protocol which aims to achieve and maintain compensation can be performed. The exercises are subdivided according to different phases of equilibrium, from supine to standing to moving. In each part, there is a progression from mechanics to synergetics exercises. The exercises aim to enable the patient to achieve compensation at home as far as possible, reducing secondary damage and avoiding tertiary damage. The complete protocol must be initially performed twice a day for 10 days. After this period the protocol can be reduced to the following exercises, to be performed twice a day for at least 1 month: 8, 14, 19, 21, 22, 23, 28, 33.

A. Supine
1. Hold your knee which is the opposite site of the lesion against the chest, then extend your leg. When you hold your knee against the chest with the hands, gently apply traction to the flexed leg (Fig. 4.37).
2. Take your arm which is the same side as the lesion, extend it over your head and simultaneously hold the contralateral flexed leg to your chest, using your hand for assistance. Maintain this position for 10 s (Fig. 4.38).
3. Lift your leg on the same side as the lesion with the knee extended (Fig. 4.39).
4. Repeat with the tip of the foot outward.
5. Repeat with the tip of the foot inward.

Fig. 4.37. Patient holds
the knee against the chest

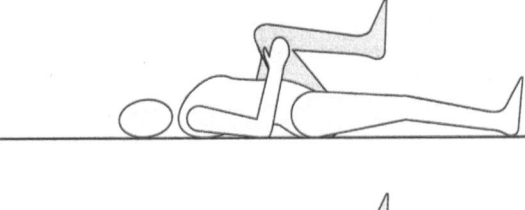

Fig. 4.38. Patient extends
the arm on the affected
side and at the same time
holds the opposite knee
against the chest

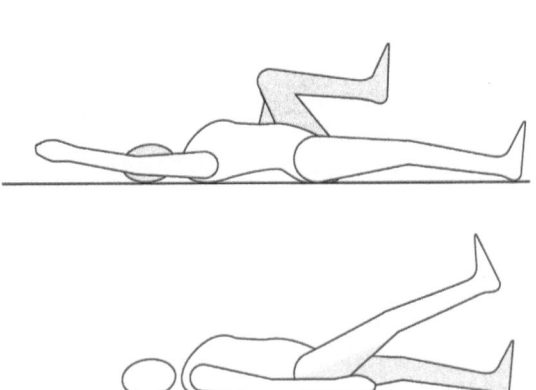

Fig. 4.39. Extension of
the leg on the affected
side

6. Put a pillow under your leg (on the same side as the lesion). Bind a 2-kg weight to your ankle with the knee flexed; then extend it.
7. Lift your pelvis and simultaneously extend your arms over your head. Then drop your arms back along your body and lower your pelvis (Fig. 4.40).
8. Turn your head toward the side of lesion and fixate a target on the lateral wall. Then straighten your head straight while maintaining the visual fixation. Count up to 10 and then turn your head.
9. From the supine position move to the sitting position while fixating a point straight in front of you.
10. In the prone position lift your left arm and right leg, maintaining your forehead over the bed. Then repeat the maneuver with the right arm and the left leg (Fig. 4.41).
11. Repeat as above but simultaneously lifting also the head.
B. Sitting
12. Extend your right arm and lift your thumb. Move your arm slowly to and fro first in a horizontal direction and then in a vertical direction. Follow your thumb with the eyes only, first slowly and then progressively increasing the velocity of thumb displacement.
13. As above but simultaneously moving also the head while trying to keep the eyes still.

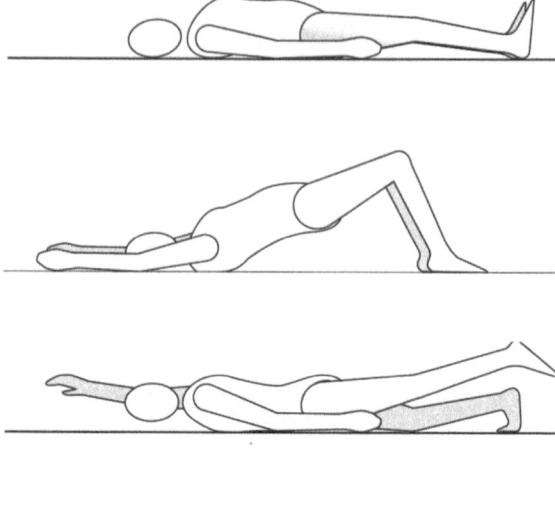

Fig. 4.40. Patient extends the arms lifting the pelvis

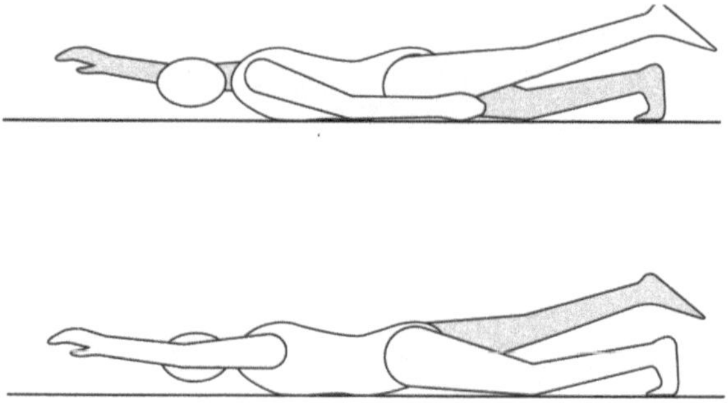

Fig. 4.41. Patient extends the right arm and left leg, in the prone position and then alternates the arm and leg

14. Open a book in front of you. Read it moving, simultaneously, the book right and left and then to and fro.

C. Standing

15. With your hands on a table lift yourself onto your tiptoes with your weight on the leg on the same side as the lesion; maintain this position for 30 s (Fig. 4.42).

16. With your hands on a table lift yourself onto your heels, with your weight on the leg on the same side as the lesion; maintain this position for 30 s (Fig. 4.43).

17. Fixate your image in a mirror. Align your position correctly. Maintain equilibrium for 1 min and then close your eyes and continue visualizing your correct position; remain in this position for at least 1 min (Fig. 4.44).

18. Repeat the same exercise standing on a soft mattress.

19. Hold a small object and then lift it over your head and fixate it. With your extended arms move it in circles of increasing width while maintaining your fixation of the object (Fig. 4.45).

20. Repeat the same exercise with the eyes closed.

21. Repeat the exercise again standing on a soft mattress.

Fig. 4.42. Patient lifts himself standing on tiptoes

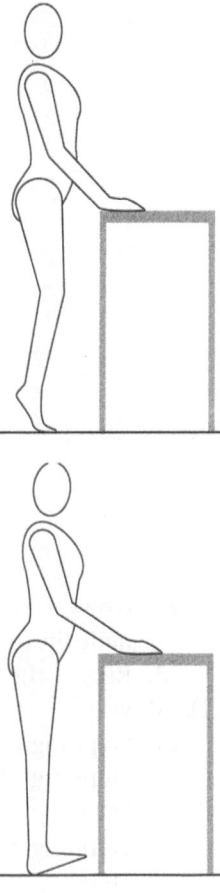

Fig. 4.43. As above but standing on the heels

Fig. 4.44. Facing a mirror, the patient aligns himself correctly and then closes his eyes maintaining a correct posture

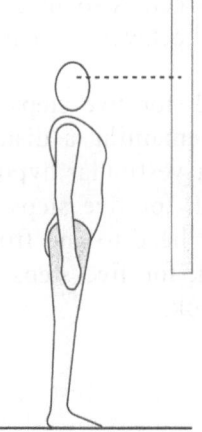
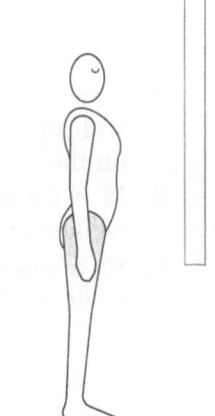

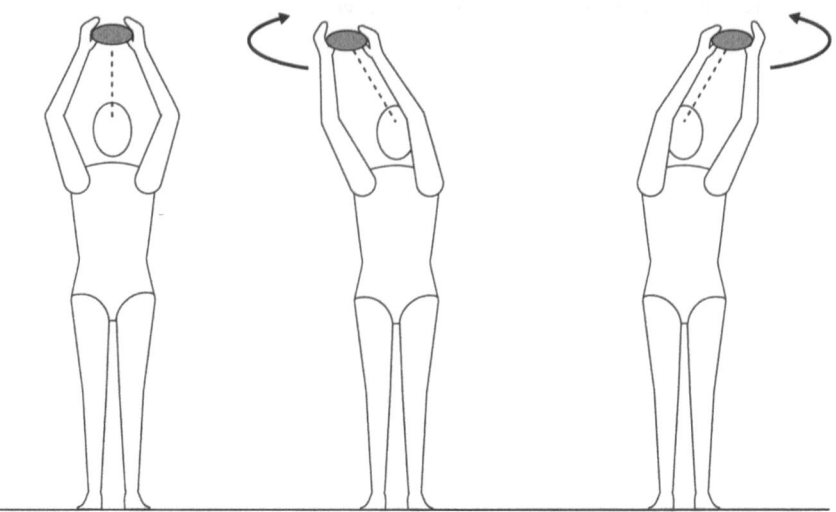

Fig. 4.45. Patient moves an object in circles while fixating it

22. Open a book in front of you. Read it while moving it simultaneously to and fro and from side to side.
23. Repeat the same exercise on a soft mattress.
D. Moving
24. Stepping on the floor with eyes open.
25. Stepping while fixating a target in front of you.
26. Stepping with eyes closed.
27. Stepping moving the head to and fro.
28. Stepping while reading a book.
29. In a corridor, walk for five steps forward and then backward while fixating a target. Also in a corridor, walk for five steps forward and then backward staring, without any reference target.
30. In a corridor, walk for five steps forward and then backward with eyes closed remaining a distance of 20 cm from the wall on the side of your vestibular hypofunction.
31. In a corridor, walk for five steps forward and then backward while moving your head to and fro.
32. In a corridor walk for five steps forward and then backward while reading a book.

Uncompensated Unilateral Vestibular Hypofunction

Vestibular unilateral hypofunction is a consequence of the primary damage to the vestibular structures. Incorrect or incomplete compensation can cause secondary and tertiary damage. Natural compensatory phenomena require, without any kind of treatment, a period ranging from 6 to 8 months to achieve a good functional recovery. This kind of recovery is not always sufficient to allow performing even everyday life activities in a natural, unconscious and easy manner. Some activities are still difficult such as turning the head rapidly or changing positions of the body and, frequently, transient vertigo attacks and subcontinuous unsteadiness are observed. Even some years after an acute episode of vertigo, compensation can turn into transient failure and can cause either vertigo or dizziness.

Functional and instrumental evaluation must be aimed at investigating the condition of recovery mechanisms in order to evaluate whether the failure concerns the mechanics, cybernetics or synergetics aspects of the equilibrium system.

This protocol can also be adopted to treat dizziness in patients with Meniere's disease during the intercritical period. Vertigo attacks cannot be prevented by rehabilitation but often patients complain of both sporadic vertigo attacks and continuous unsteadiness. This condition can be treated as a vestibular unilateral hypofunction.

Rehabilitation is the specific treatment of unilateral vestibular hypofunction. In fact even when the etiology of hypofunction is known, as after the operation of neurinoma, after an attack of neuronitis, with postconcussion syndrome or even when viral or vascular etiology is supposed or confirmed, improvement of the dizziness cannot always be obtained by acting upon these etiologic factors, or by administration of some symptomatic drugs. In all these cases with unilateral hypofunction, only the phenomena of the central regulation – the compensation – is able to render these patients free from dizziness. Thus it is of the utmost importance to stimulate these physiological mechanisms in order to abolish the dizzy spells. In many cases, it is the only way to treat them.

Treatment must be aim to:
1. Increase extensory tone on the affected side.
2. Increase antigravitational paravertebral tone.
3. Restore correct ankle/hip dynamic strategies.
4. Restore control of head stabilization during movement.
5. Restore eye/head coordination.
6. Avoid disorientation attacks (vertigo attacks).

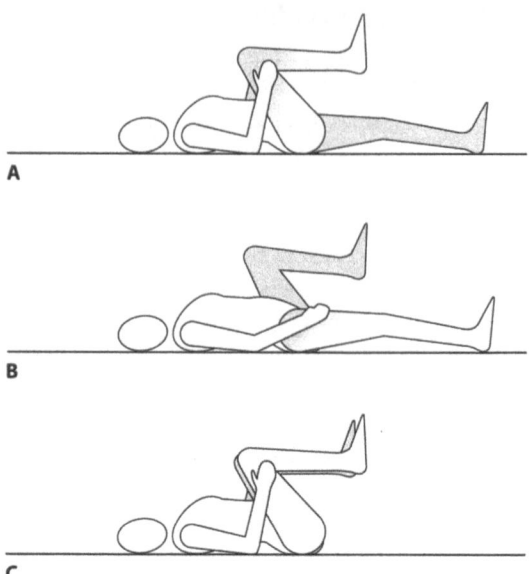

Fig. 4.46A–C. Exercises holding the knees against the chest

A

B

C

Exercises in the Gymnasium

Mechanics Phase

1. Relaxation exercises such as control of breathing with improving consciousness of the abdomen or thoracic breathing. A simple exercise consists of a deep inhalation followed, after a few seconds, by a forced exhalation pronouncing the word "one." This exercise is repeated 8–10 times.
2. The patient holds his right knee against the chest, then extends his leg and holds his left knee against the chest. When he holds the knee against the chest he gently applies traction to the flexed leg with the hands (Fig. 4.46A, B).
3. The patient holds his two knees to the chest while simultaneously helping, gently, with the hands (Fig. 4.46C).
4. With the flexed legs and the feet on the bed, the patient rotates his pelvis rightward and leftward keeping his knees flexed and his legs together (Fig. 4.47).
5. The patient lifts his pelvis while simultaneously holding his arms extended over his head. He then repositions his arms along the body while lowering the pelvis (Fig. 4.48).
6. In the quadrupedal position the patient inhales and arches his back (hyperkyphosis) while holding his head between his arms.

Fig. 4.47. Rotation of the pelvis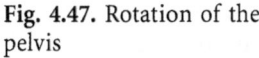

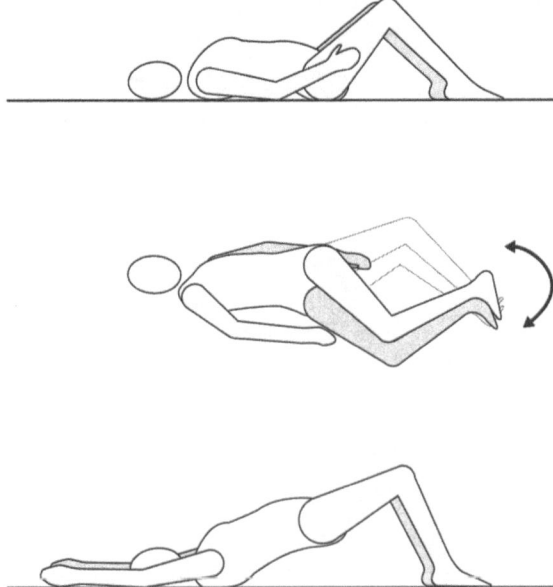

Fig. 4.48. Patient lifts the pelvis and then returns to the supine position

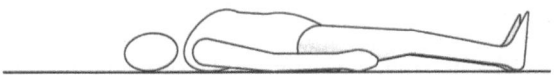

He then exhales, flexing the head and rotating the pelvis in hyperlordosis (Fig. 4.49).

7. From the supine position the patient passes to the sitting position fixating a point straight in front of him (Fig. 4.50).

8. The patient, with a pillow under the leg (by the affected side) and with a 2-kg weight bound to the ankle, extends the leg (Fig. 4.51).

Meniere's Disease

In the sitting position the patient grasps a stick with both hands and takes the stick behind his shoulder positioning the stick at the level of the cervicodorsal junction. In this position he pushes the stick against his back exhaling and inhaling rhythmically and slowly. He then repeats the exercise moving the stick forward on the sternum at the level of the sternoclavicular joint. The patient grasps the stick with the hands frontally positioned.

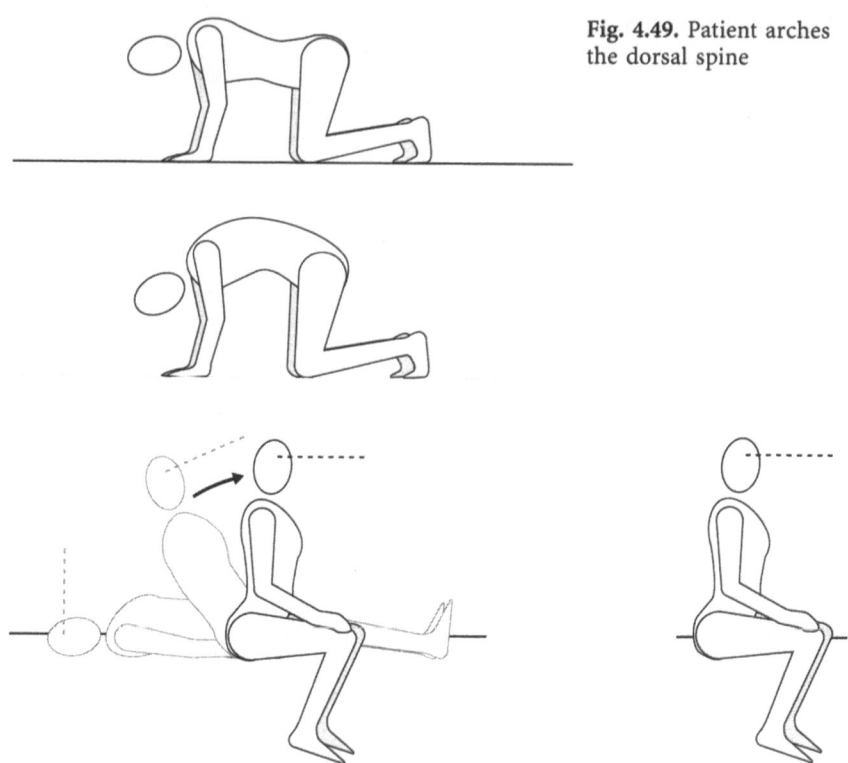

Fig. 4.49. Patient arches the dorsal spine

Fig. 4.50. From the supine to the sitting position fixating a target

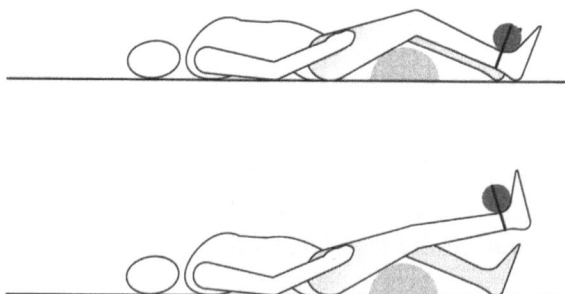

Fig. 4.51. With a weight bound to the ankle the patient extends the leg on the affected side

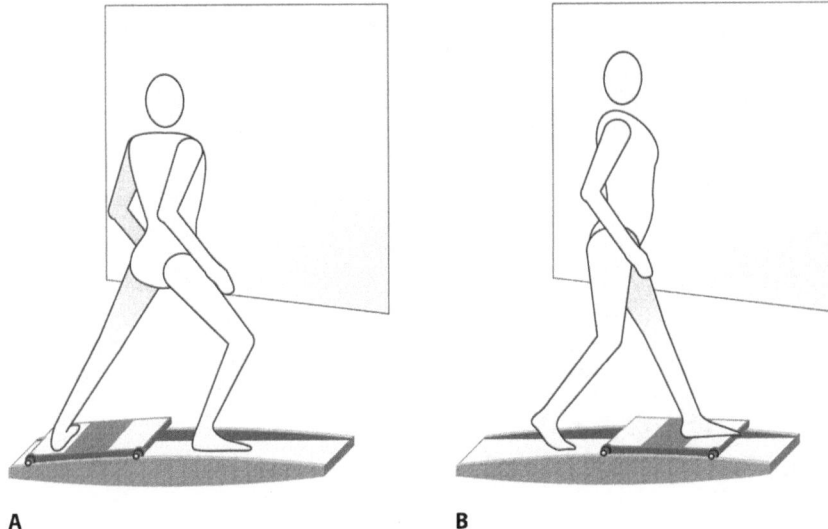

A   **B**

Fig. 4.52. A Backward extension of the leg; **B** forward extension of the leg

9. On the Skitter, looking at a mirror:
   a) With one foot on the end cap and the other across the footpad, the patient keeps his weight backward and extends the leg on the side of the lesion in a controlled manner, then returning slowly and repeating. The patient then performs leg extension with closed eyes to improve self-perception of muscle tone (Fig. 4.52A).
   b) Similar to above except the focus is on the front leg. With a stable, controlled movement, the patient extends the end of the leg forward (Fig. 4.52B).

Cybernetics Phase
These exercises have to be performed during vestibular electrical stimulation (VES), placing the electrodes on the trapezius of the affected side and the paravertebral muscles of the opposite side.
10. Using the Skitter, looking at a mirror
    a) With one foot on the end cap and the other across the footpad, the patient keeps his weight forward and extends the front leg, on the side of the affected labyrinth. The patient maintains the leg extension position and the therapist destabilizes him moving the platform during visual fixation of a target (see Fig. 4.52A).
    b) The patient performs backward leg extensions. With a stable, controlled movement, the patient extends the leg back to the

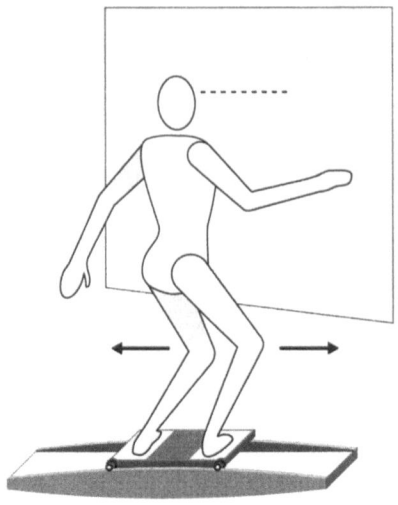

Fig. 4.53. Patient moves his weight to and fro fixating himself in a mirror

end, then maintaining the leg extension position, and the therapist destabilizes him by moving the platform during visual fixation (see Fig. 4.52B).

c) The patient steps on the footpads with feet centrally positioned. He then concentrates on a proper posture using a mirror to see his reflection and transfers his weight from one foot to the other with a smooth flowing motion. During this smooth and rhythmic weight transfer the therapist induces body movements according to ankle or hip strategies (Fig. 4.53).

d) The patient is comfortably stable on the footpads. With his thumbs and extended limbs he tries to touch visual targets placed in different positions on a facing mirror (Fig. 4.54).

e) The patient maintains equilibrium on one leg (on the affected side) with the other leg laterally positioned. The therapist helps the patient either maintain equilibrium or to correct his posture. A mirror facilitates the correction of the postural equilibrium strategy. Visual prisms (3–5°) based on the opposite side of the lesion help increase the extensory activity of the muscle on the same side of the lesion (Fig. 4.55).

11. Using the Rettiks mattress

a) The patient wearing prisms fixates himself in a mirror. The therapist helps him to align his position correctly. He must maintain equilibrium for 1 min with eyes open and then close his eyes and visualize his correct position while remaining in this position for at least 1 min.

Fig. 4.54. The patient stands on the Skitter and has to point to different targets placed on a mirror

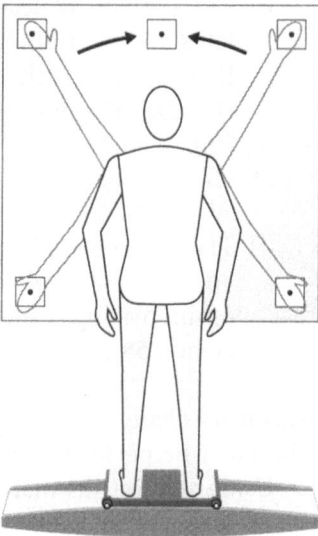

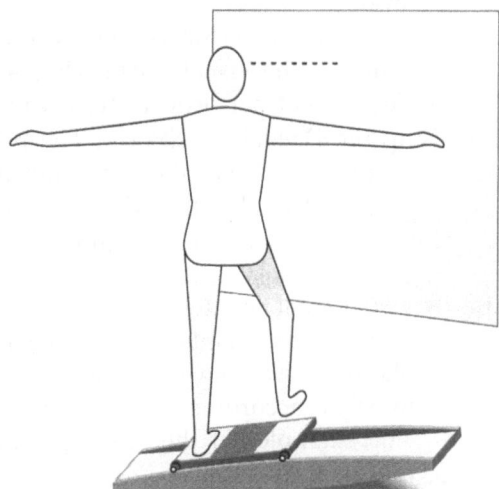

Fig. 4.55. The patient fixates himself in a mirror and maintains equilibrium standing on the leg on the affected side

b) The patient fixates himself in a mirror (Fig. 4.56A), then oscillates to the right and left (Fig. 4.56B) around his pelvis. He then resists the therapist's attempts at destabilization (Fig. 4.56C) and maintains equilibrium while crossing the legs (Fig. 4.56D).

c) The patient oscillates to and fro around his ankles while maintaining fixation in a mirror (Fig. 4.57).

d) The patient holds a small object and then lifts it over his head and fixates it. With his extended arms, he moves it in circles of increasing width while maintaining fixation of the object (Fig. 4.58).

Synergetics Phase

VES must be performed also during the exercises of this phase.

12. Using the Rettiks mattress

a) The patient opens a book in front of him and then moves it away from him extending his arms. He reads it then moves it closer to him, slowly, while trying to read it. Then he moves it away.

b) The patient performs steps while fixating a target in front of him wearing visual prisms (Fig. 4.59).

c) The patient performs a steps while reading a book.

13. Using the Daedalus platform: The patient stands on the table and tries to maneuver the ball through the complete labyrinth (Fig. 4.60). He takes the sticks that have to be placed in the posterior holes in order to improve extensory posterior activity (Fig. 4.61).

14. By visual-feedback devices

a) The patient stands in a stable position on the stabilometric platform, wearing no shoes. The position of the visual targets must be according to the side of the lesion. In Figs. 4.62 and 4.63 examples of the target position for right vestibular hypofunction are shown.

b) The patient is stable on the platform, with shoes on, and wearing a lift heel on the same side of lesion. The position of the targets is the same.

15. Moving

a) The patient walks five steps forward and backward fixating a target, wearing prisms.

b) The patient walks five steps forward and backward with eyes closed remaining a distance of 20 cm from the wall on the side of his vestibular hypofunction.

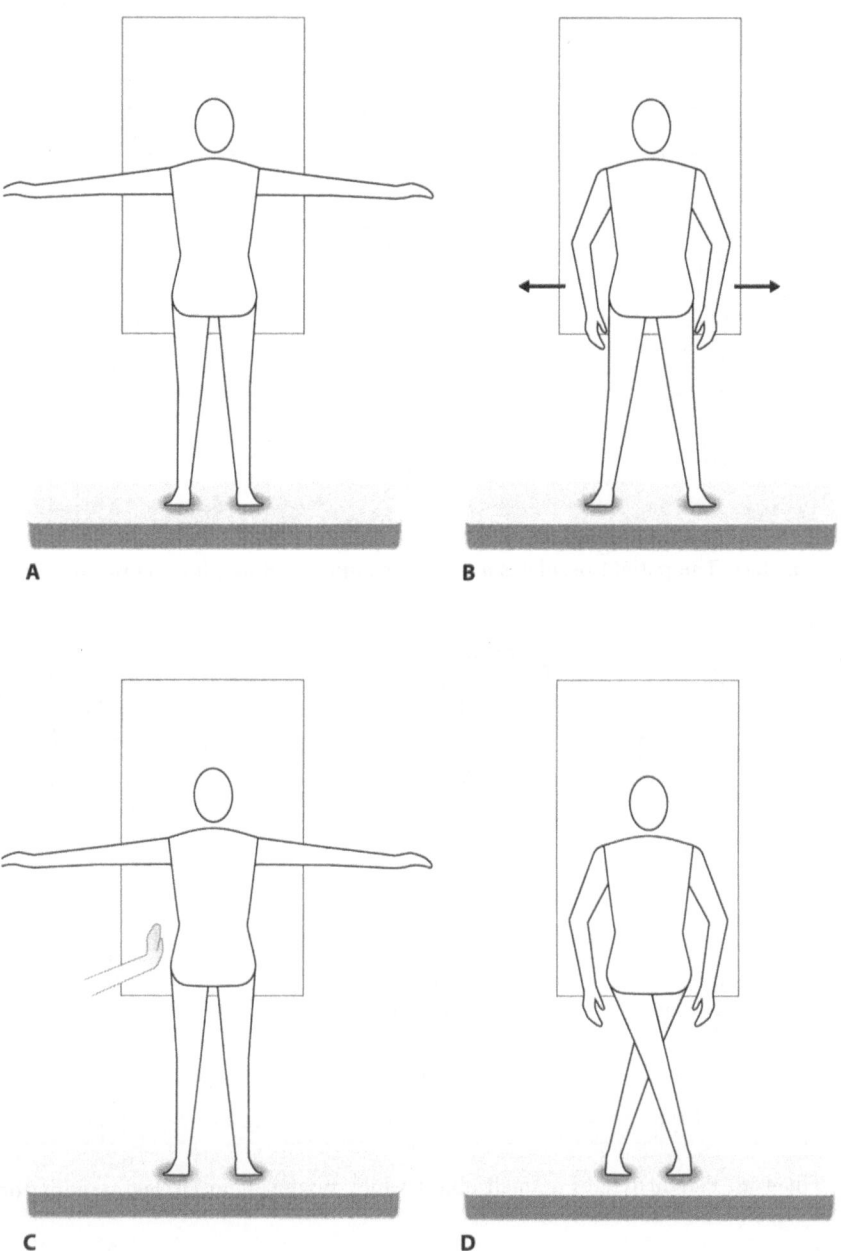

Fig. 4.56. The patient aligns himself looking at a mirror (**A**), then he oscillates (**B**), then resists when the therapist destabilizes him (**C**) or he maintains equilibrium crossing the legs (**D**)

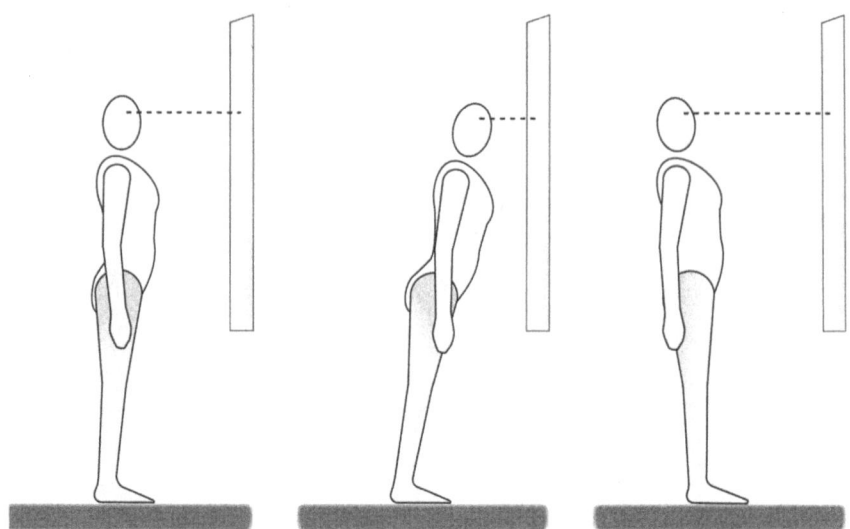

Fig. 4.57. The patient oscillates around his ankles maintaining the pelvis still

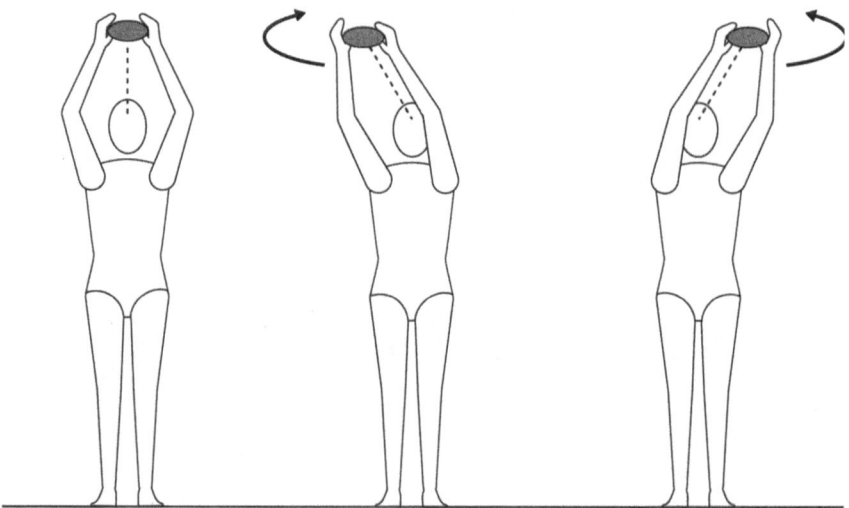

Fig. 4.58. Patient fixates a small object while moving it in circles, standing on a mattress

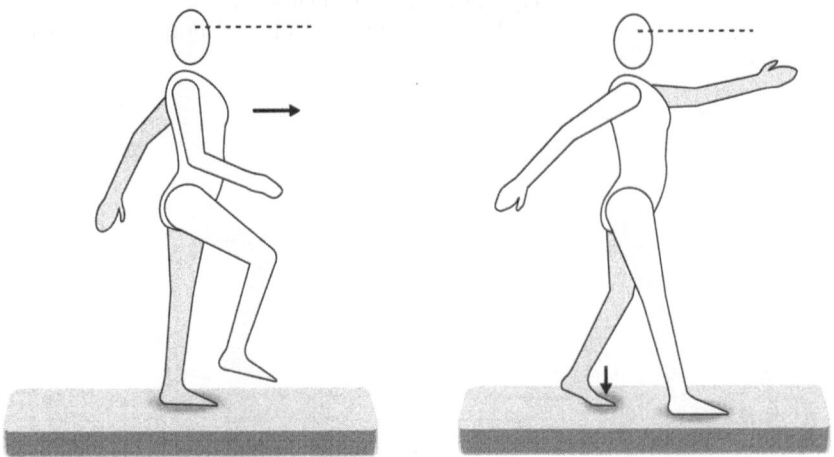

Fig. 4.59. Stepping on a mattress without and with simultaneous oscillations of the arms, fixating a target

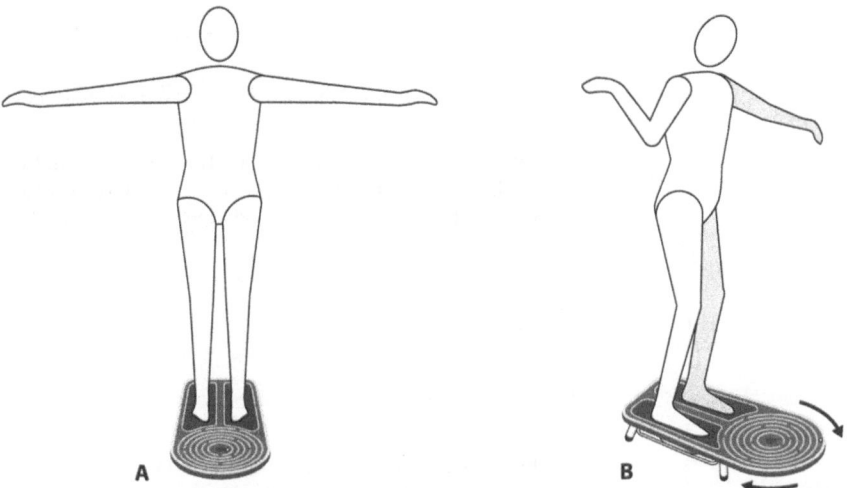

Fig. 4.60. Patient maneuvers a ball through the labyrinth

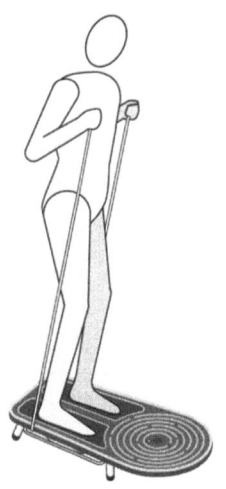

Fig. 4.61. Patient maneuvers a ball through the labyrinth grasping the sticks placed in the posterior holes

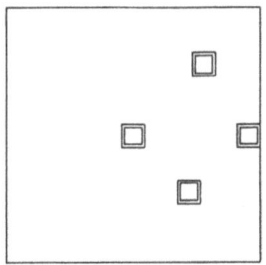

Fig. 4.62. Training for right vestibular hypofunction (Balance Master, reproduced by courtesy of NeuroCom International, Inc., Clackamas, Oregon, USA)

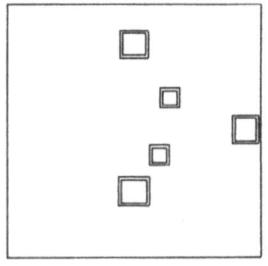

Fig. 4.63. Improving ankle-hip strategies in right hypofunction (Balance Master, reproduced by courtesy of NeuroCom International, Inc., Clackamas, Oregon, USA)

c) The patient walks five steps forward and backward moving his head to and fro, wearing prisms.

Home Protocol

The aim of the home protocol is to maintain the results obtained by the therapist. The exercises have been subdivided according to the sequence of equilibrium. Only the most effective exercises have been included in this protocol because the patient needs to repeat them twice or three times a day.

A. Supine
 1. Lift the leg on the same side of lesion with the knee extended.
 2. Repeat the exercise with the tip of the foot outward.
 3. Repeat the exercise again with the tip of the foot inward.
 4. Place a pillow under your leg (on the same side as the lesion). Bind a 2-kg weight to your ankle with the flexed knee; then extend it alternating between right and left legs.
 5. Lift your pelvis simultaneously extending your arms over your head. Then reposition your arms along the body lowering your pelvis.
 6. From the supine position pass to the sitting position, fixating a point straight ahead.

B. Sitting
 7. Extend your right arm and lift your thumb. Move your arm slowly to and fro first in a horizontal direction and then in a vertical direction. Follow your thumb with the eyes only, first slowly and then increasing progressively the velocity of thumb displacement.
 8. As above but simultaneously moving also the head while trying to keep the eyes still.
 9. Look for three targets sited, respectively, in front of you, on your left and on your right. Fixate the frontal target, then move your head rapidly fixating the right-hand target. Now turn your head leftward while maintaining the fixation of the right-hand target. Fixate the frontal target. Now rapidly move your head leftward and fixate the left-hand target. Then turn your head rightward maintaining the fixation of the left-hand target.
 10. Extend your right arm and lift your thumb. Move your arm slowly to and fro first in a horizontal direction and then in a vertical direction. Follow your thumb with the eyes only, first slowly and then increasing progressively the velocity of thumb displacement.

11. As above but moving simultaneously also the head while trying to keep the eyes still.

C. Standing

12. Standing on a soft mattress fixate your reflection in a mirror. Align your position correctly. Maintain equilibrium for 1 min, close your eyes and visualize your correct position; remain in this position for at least 1 min.

13. Hold a small object and then lift it over your head and fixate it. With your extended arms move it in circles of increasing width while maintaining the fixation of the object. Then close your eyes and continue making the circles.

14. Standing on a soft mattress open a book in front of you. Read it while simultaneously moving it to and fro and from side to side.

D. Moving

15. Stepping with eyes closed.

16. Stepping moving the head to and fro.

17. In a corridor walk for five steps forward and backward with eyes closed remaining a distance of 20 cm from the wall on the side of your vestibular hypofunction.

Paroxysmal Positional Vertigo

Paroxismal positional vertigo (PPV) is a common complaint and represents one of the most common entities in peripheral vestibular pathology. It was described by Barany in 1907 but it received its definite clinical description in the report of Dix in 1976.

The principal complaint is the occurrence of sudden attacks of vertigo precipitated by certain head positions. The attacks can be induced by rolling over in bed, to one side or to either side, by sudden movement of the head, extending the neck, looking upwards, as in reaching for an object from the top shelf in the kitchen, bending the head backwards for hair washing, lying down beneath a car or throwing the head backwards to paint a ceiling. The patient sometimes recognizes that the onset of the vertigo is associated with this critical position and will say he does his best to avoid it.

The initial occurrence is usually experienced on awakening in the morning, which is considered characteristic, or during the night. Many patients are frightened by the intense vertigo and try to shut out the sensation by closing their eyes. Nausea, often accompanied by anxiety, even vomiting, may follow the attack in a few cases. In rare cases the nausea persists for hours. Vertigo is of short duration

(<1 min) but, because of the intensity of the vertiginous sensation, a longer duration can be assigned to the attack.

Generally speaking, two main kinds of PPV can be recognized:

1. The most frequent is elicited by the so-called Dix-Hallpike maneuver that induces a typical horizontal-rotatory geotropic nystagmus while the patient is supine during simultaneous rotation and hyperextension of the head. Nystagmus appears several seconds after the execution of the maneuver (latency) and it decreases on the subsequent repetition of the same maneuver (fatigability due to habituation phenomena).

2. Vertigo and pure horizontal nystagmus are provoked by rolling the head from side to side while the patient is recumbent. In this case (MacClure's maneuver) two kinds of nystagmus can be observed, geotropic and ageotropic nystagmus.

While the clinical picture is well known and widely described, the etiopathogenesis of PPV can be considered still debatable. The most accepted theory is the lithiasis theory, originally described by Schucknecht (1974), who named the process *cupolithiasis*. According to this theory, then generally accepted, substances having a specific gravity greater than the endolymph, and thus subject to movement with changes in the direction of gravitational forces, come into contact with the cupola of the posterior semicircular canal (in the case of vertigo induced by the Dix-Hallpike maneuver) or of the lateral semicircular canal (in the case of vertigo elicited by MacClure's maneuver). The change in position of the labyrinth during movement of the head provokes the displacement of the cupola by direct influence of these heavy substances on it. Recently cupolithiasis has been discussed and the theory of free-floating particles in the canal (so-called *canalolithiasis)* has been formulated.

On the basis of these theories, maneuvers aimed at the "liberation" of the cupola or the canal from floating particles have been proposed. The two main ones are Semont's and Epley's maneuvers. They differ in movement and in rapidity but they are both effective in at least 80%–90% of the patients affected with the most frequent so-called lithiasis of the posterior semicircular canal, after one or two single treatment sessions. For the least frequent so-called horizontal semicircular canal lithiasis, Lempert proposed an effective maneuver.

Lithiasis theories are still controversial because they are not able to explain all the features of PPV, especially when the proposed maneuvers are not effective or when the signs and symptoms are not as typical as those described above (about 10% of the patients suffering positional vertigo). Another explanation considers the otoliths as the source of nystagmus, but in the sense of influencing and favoring a nystagmus primarily elicited by the canals. Emphasis is upon the otolith-canal interaction. According to Ledouz, the vertical canals and the utricles form a system of sensory organs which function synergically. The system of the contralateral side has an antagonistic function. Asymmetry in this coupling can bring about a disturbing situation, i.e., vertigo and nystagmus. Some authors proposed that central mechanisms are involved. Ledoux argued that the modalities of appearance of PPV can only occur through a modification in the central channels of the equilibrium normally existing between the influxes of both labyrinths. This rupture is checked by an inhibition phenomenon during the attack or during repeated provocation. McCabe explained PPV as the result of focal microscopic loss of otolithic macular epithelium by either a neurovirus or a microstroke.

According to MCS concepts, positional vertigo can be interpreted as a *proprioceptive mismatch* between the so-called general proprioception (from muscle, ligaments and joints) and the so-called special proprioception (from maculae and cristae) according to the spinocerebello-vestibulospinal circuitry described by Drukker (Fig. 4.64), which means that these different items of proprioceptive information are integrated and elaborated in the cerebellum and then projected on the vestibular nuclei.

Despite the different interpretation of PPV etiopathogenesis, the effectiveness of the maneuvers described by Semont, Epley and Lempert and their modifications is without doubt. For this reason the first therapeutic approach must be by means of one of these treatments.

Semont's Maneuver

The patient lies on the affected side for at least 3 min (in Fig. 4.65A a left PPV is represented). Then the head is rotated upward about 105° (in the cupolithiasis theory) in order to allow the displacement of the heavy particles at the basis of the posterior semicircular canal with downward deflection of the cupola. Then the therapist takes firmly the head of the patient (Fig. 4.65B) and decisively brings the patient onto the opposite side with a simultaneous rotation of the head downward about 195° (Fig. 4.65C). Usually, in this position, after few seconds, a "liberating" nystagmus toward the affected side appears. When nystagmus and vertigo disappear, the patient returns slowly to the sitting position.

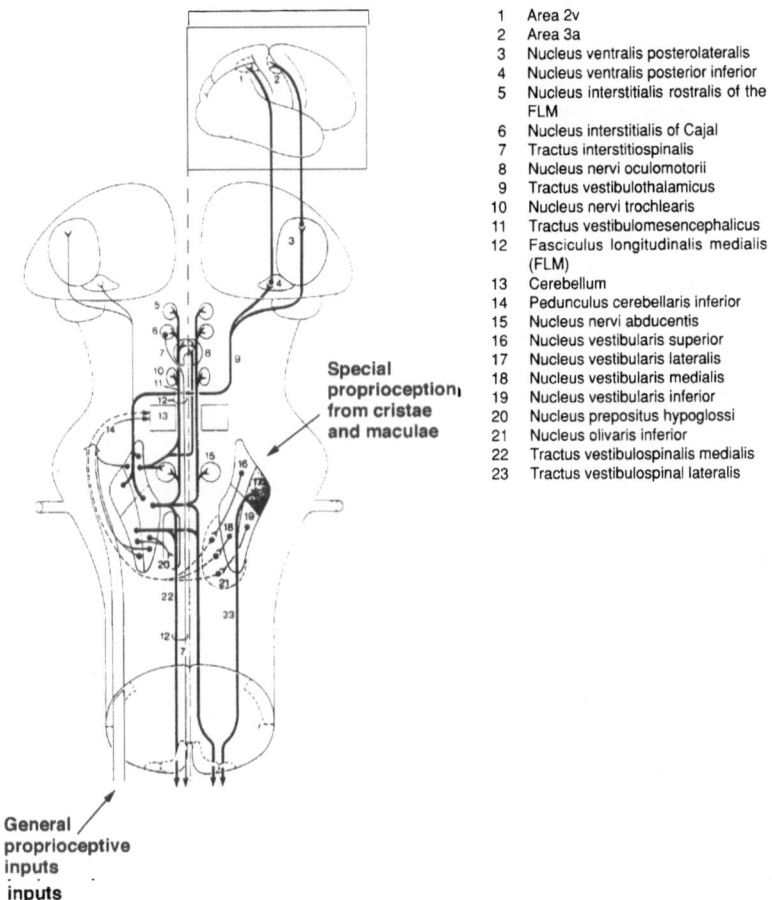

1   Area 2v
2   Area 3a
3   Nucleus ventralis posterolateralis
4   Nucleus ventralis posterior inferior
5   Nucleus interstitialis rostralis of the
    FLM
6   Nucleus interstitialis of Cajal
7   Tractus interstitiospinalis
8   Nucleus nervi oculomotorii
9   Tractus vestibulothalamicus
10 Nucleus nervi trochlearis
11 Tractus vestibulomesencephalicus
12 Fasciculus longitudinalis medialis
    (FLM)
13 Cerebellum
14 Pedunculus cerebellaris inferior
15 Nucleus nervi abducentis
16 Nucleus vestibularis superior
17 Nucleus vestibularis lateralis
18 Nucleus vestibularis medialis
19 Nucleus vestibularis inferior
20 Nucleus prepositus hypoglossi
21 Nucleus olivaris inferior
22 Tractus vestibulospinalis medialis
23 Tractus vestibulospinal lateralis

Special
proprioception₁
from cristae
and maculae

General
proprioceptive
inputs
inputs

Fig. 4.64. Correlation between general and special proprioception, according to Drukker, showing the connections of the vestibular system: efferent connections of the vestibular nuclei and the spinocerebello-vestibulospinal circuitry

Epley's Maneuver

According to the original description of the technique, the patient is premedicated with transdermal scopolamine the night before, or diazepam 5 mg. The patient is seated on an examining table (Fig. 4.66A) so that when the patient is brought to the supine position, the head extends beyond the neck. The operator is located directly behind the patient, with an assistant at the patient's side. Throughout the positioning maneuvers, oscillations of the skull are optionally induced. The hand-held oscillator of the Swedish type with a frequency of approximately 80 Hz does not actually touch the head but acts through

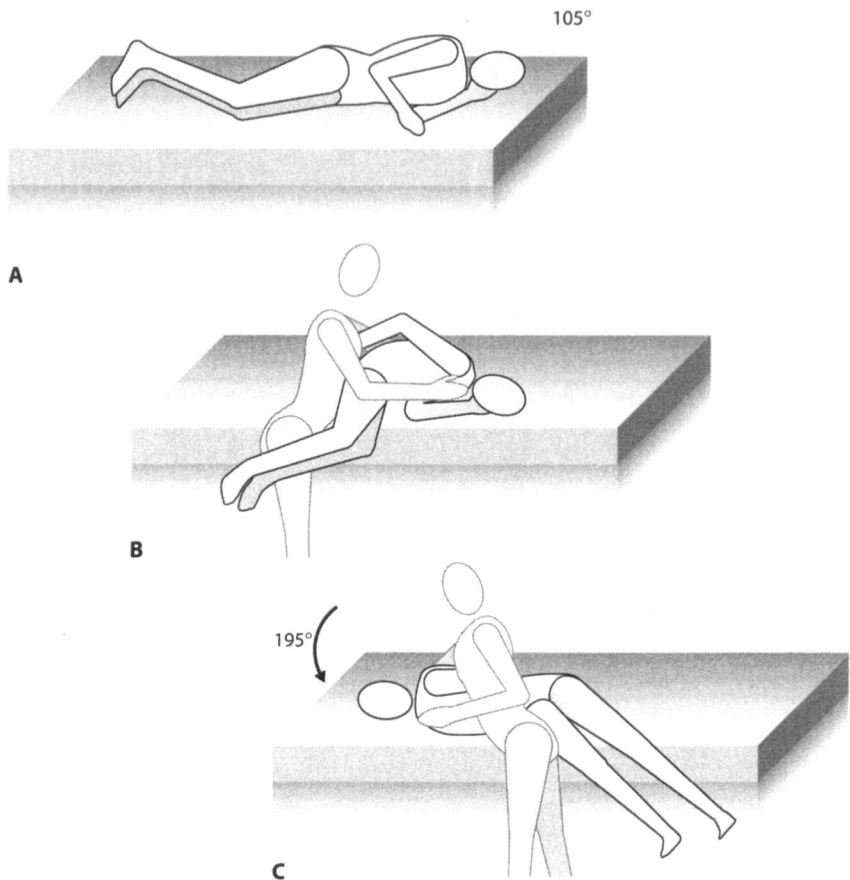

Fig. 4.65A–C. Semont's maneuver

the operator's hand applied to the ipsilateral mastoid process. The patient then lies downward with a slight hyperextension of the head and a simultaneous 105° rotation towards the affected side (on the left in Fig. 4.66B). In this position nystagmus and vertigo appear. The patient remains in each position for 6–13 s but this may be extended to more than 30 s. The head is then rotated by 90° onto the opposite side toward the healthy labyrinth (Fig. 4.66C). At the same time as head rotation the trunk and the legs are also rotated toward the healthy side (Fig. 4.66D). In this position, a "liberating" nystagmus is usually observed. The patient completes the rotation of the legs and returns to a sitting position keeping the head turned toward the opposite side with respect to the affected labyrinth (Fig. 4.66E).

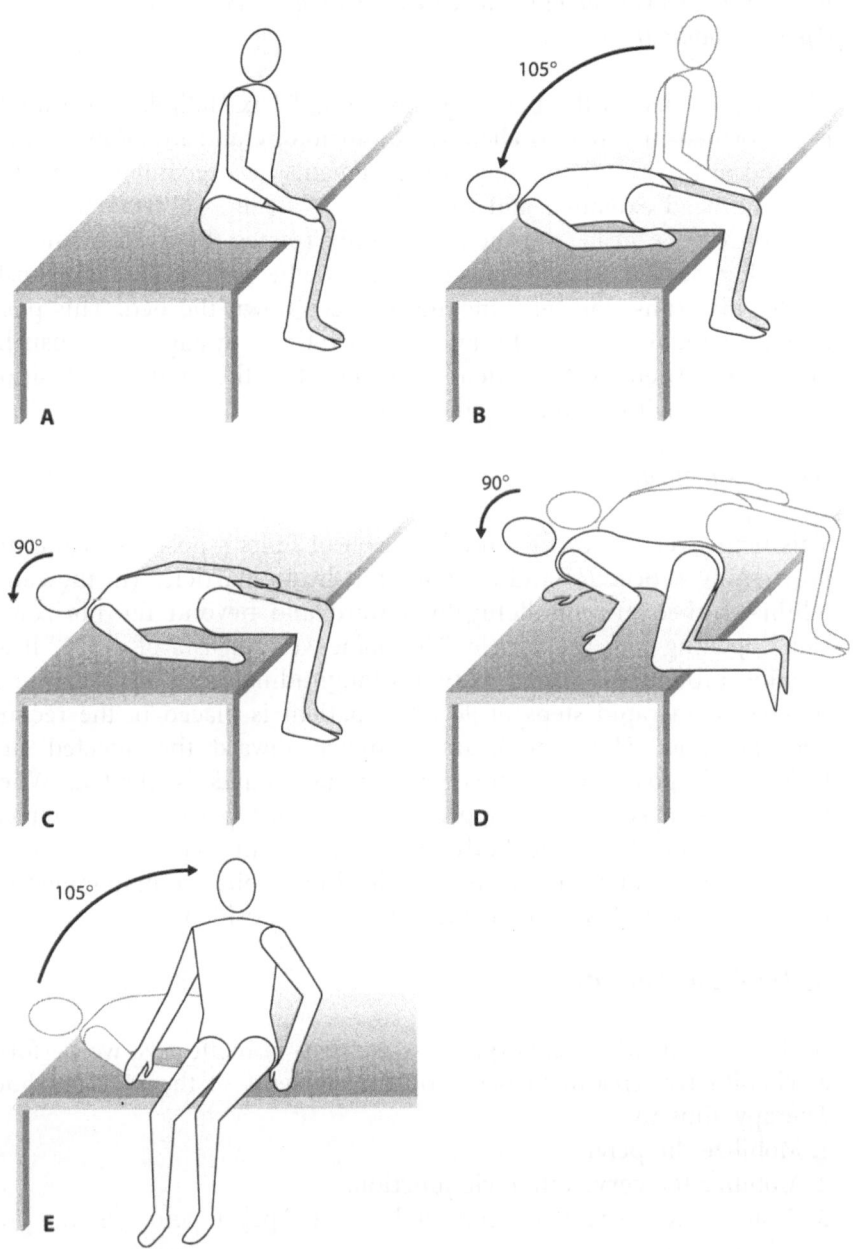

Fig. 4.66A–E. Epley's maneuver

Personal Maneuver for PPV Elicited by Dix-Hallpike Positioning (Epley's Modified)

The patient sits on the bed (Fig. 4.67A) and Dix-Hallpike positioning is performed in order to elicit symptomatology and nystagmus. After the end of the nystagmus the patient remains in a recumbent position with the head extended and rotated for 30 s (Fig. 4.67B). With slight traction on the head, the therapist gently rotates the head of the patient (Fig. 4.67C) to the opposite side and the patient simultaneously rotates his trunk and legs, moving his legs down the bed. This position is maintained for 30 s and a "liberating" nystagmus is usually observed. Then the patient returns to the sitting position (Fig. 4.67D), without turning the head.

Lempert's Maneuver

This maneuver represents an adaptation of Epley's posterior canal repositioning procedure and aims to shift heavy particles (in the canalolithiasis theory) ampullofugally toward and beyond the horizontal canal opening into the utricle. The maneuver consists of a 270° head rotation around the supine patient's longitudinal axis; the rotation is performed in rapid steps of 90°. The patient is placed in the recumbent position. Then the head is rotated toward the affected side (MacClure's position). In this position nystagmus is elicited. When vertigo and nystagmus disappear, the therapist performs a complete rotation of the head and body of the patient in steps of 90° until a complete 270° rotation is achieved. Head positions are maintained for between 30 and 60 s until all nystagmus has subsided.

No Resolution Patients

In the cases in which this type of treatment is ineffective we perform a rehabilitative treatment based on the concepts of the MCS method. Therapy aims to:
1. Mobilize the pelvis.
2. Mobilize the cervicothoracic junction.
3. Restore the correct integration between special and general proprioception.
4. Restore the correct internal representation of posture.

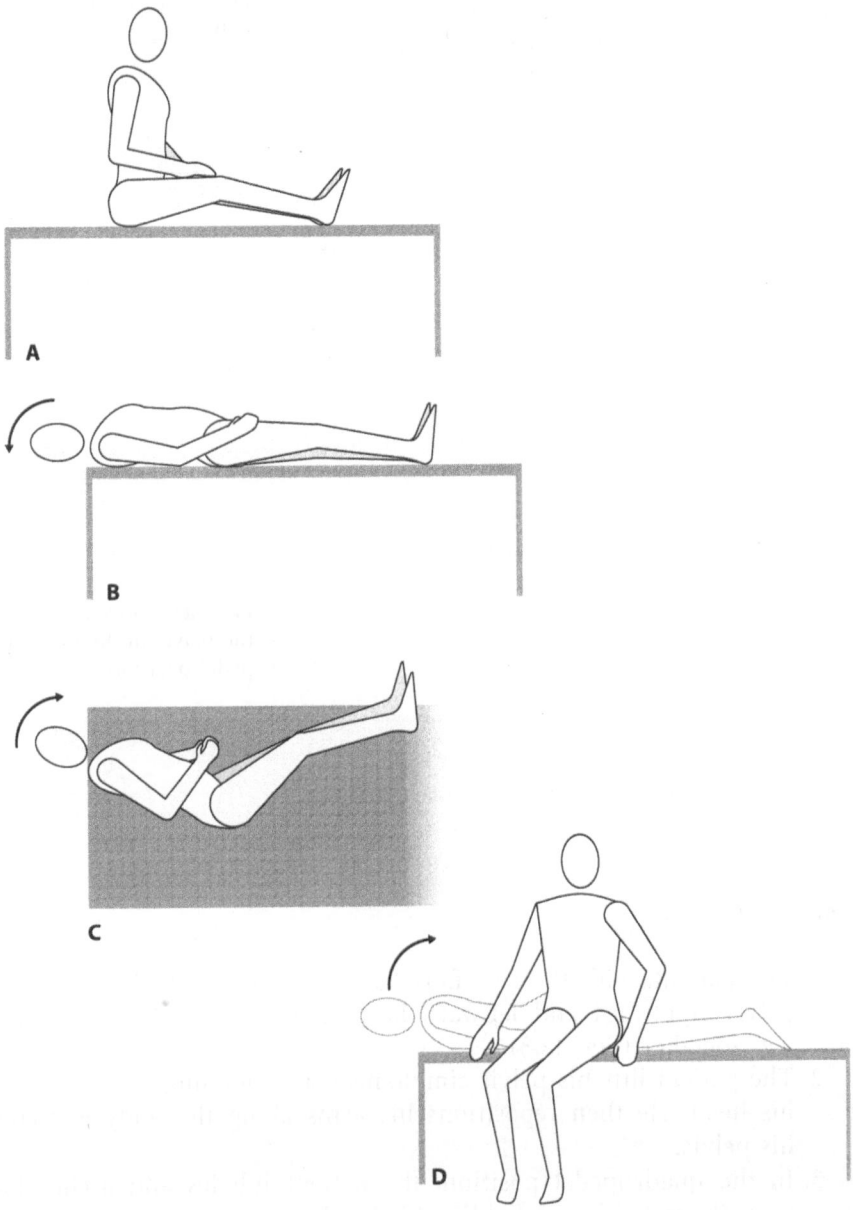

Fig. 4.67A–D. Personal maneuver for positional vertigo

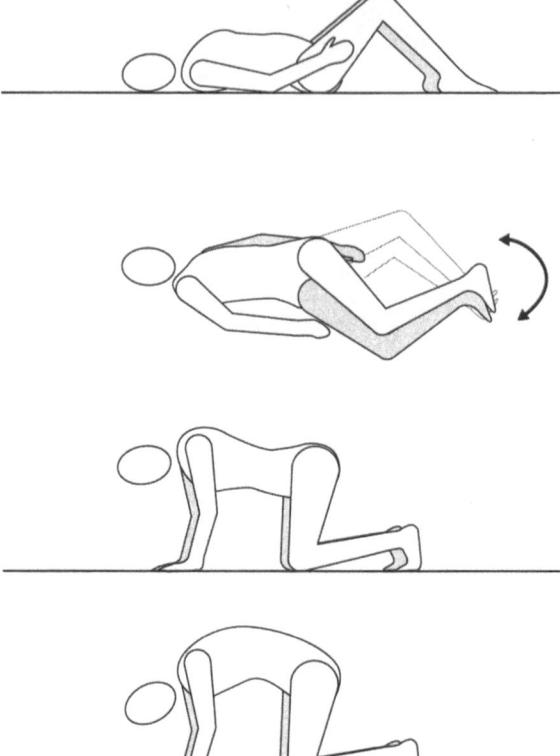

Fig. 4.68. Rotation of the pelvis

Fig. 4.69. Movements of the pelvis in the quadrupedal position

Mechanics Phase

1. The patient, with the legs flexed and feet on the bed, rotates his pelvis rightward and leftward keeping his knees flexed and his legs together (Fig. 4.68).
2. The patient lifts his pelvis simultaneously extending his arms over his head. He then repositions his arms along the body lowering his pelvis.
3. In the quadrupedal position, the patient inhales and arches his back (hyperkyphosis) holding his head between his arms. He then exhales flexing his head and rotating the pelvis in hyperlordosis (Fig. 4.69).
4. In the prone position the patient lifts his left arm and right leg while holding his forehead over the bed. He repeats the movement with the right arm and the left leg (Fig. 4.70).

Fig. 4.70. In the prone position simultaneous extension of one arm and the opposite leg

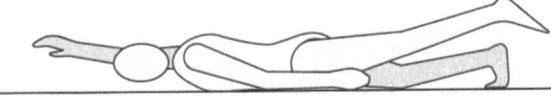

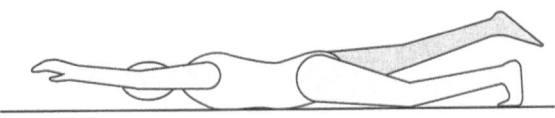

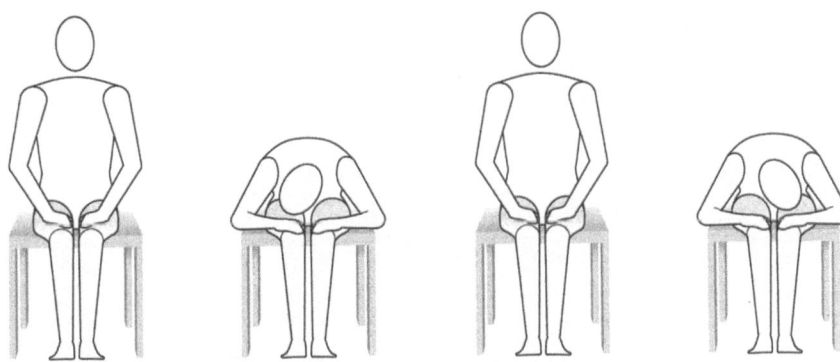

Fig. 4.71. Bending the trunk and holding the forehead on a knee

5. He repeats the procedure as above but simultaneously lifting also the head.
6. In the sitting position the patient first inhales. Then, exhaling, he bends forward holding his head on the right knee. He waits 10 s and then, inhaling, he returns to the sitting position. Then, exhaling, he bends forward holding his head on the left knee. He waits 10 s and then, inhaling, he returns to the sitting position (Fig. 4.71).
7. In the sitting position the patient grasps a stick with his hands. Then he holds it against the upper part of the sternum at the level of the sternoclavicular joint. Then, rhythmically, he performs backward displacements of the shoulders.

Cybernetics Phase

8. In the recumbent position the patient rotates his head rightward and fixates a target on the lateral wall. Then he straightens his head maintaining the visual fixation. He counts up to 10 and then rotates his head.

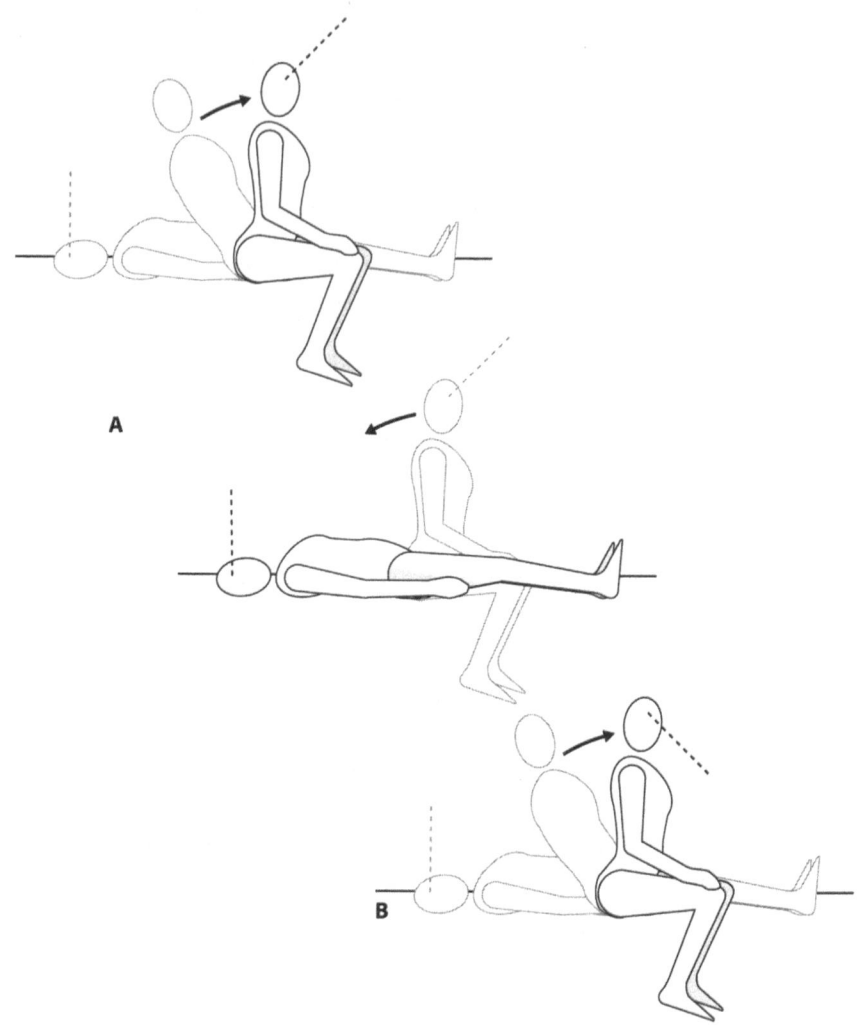

Fig. 4.72A, B. From the supine to the sitting position with simultaneous fixation of a target

9. The patient rotates his head leftward and fixates a target on the lateral wall. Then he straightens his head maintaining the visual fixation. He counts up to 10 and then rotates his head.
10. From the supine position the patient moves to the sitting position fixating a point on his left (Fig. 4.72A).
11. From the supine position the patient moves to the sitting position fixating a point on his right (Fig. 4.72B).

12. In the supine position the patient moves his head first slowly and then more rapidly in all directions fixating a target straight in front of him.

13. Sitting, the patient looks for three targets sited, respectively, in front of him, on his left and on his right. He fixates the front target, then moves rapidly his head fixating the right-hand target. Now he turns his head leftward maintaining the fixation of the right-hand target. He then fixates the front target. Now he rapidly moves his head leftward and fixates the left-hand target. Then he turns his head rightward maintaining the fixation of the left-hand target.

14. Standing, the patient holds a small object and lifts it over his head and fixates it. He inhales. Then exhaling he bends forward picking up the object on the floor. He waits 10 s and then inhaling he again lifts the object over his head.

15. The patient holds a small object and lifts it over his head while fixating it. He lifts it over his head and then, with straight arms, he moves the object in circles of increasing width and, simultaneously bending his trunk and knees, he picks it up from the floor.

16. He repeats the exercise on a soft mattress (Rettiks).

17. Using the Skitter.
    a) The patient steps on the footpads with the feet centrally positioned and concentrates on a proper posture using a mirror to see his reflection. With eyes closed he transfers his weight from one foot to the other with a smooth flowing motion. During this smooth and rhythmic weight transfer the therapist pushes the bumpers at one end of the Skitter, inducing a sudden and unpredictable inclination of the device (Fig. 4.73A).
    b) The patient steps on the footpads with the feet centrally positioned. Then he concentrates on a proper posture using a mirror to see his reflection and begins to transfer his weight from one foot to the other with a smooth flowing motion. As his rhythms increase, he moves closer to the bumpers at each end always maintaining a good upright posture with eyes focused in the mirror and paying attention to his balance. The exercise can be performed with limited upper body movement (such as in slalom) or including upper body motion (such as in giant slalom). Exercises need to be performed concentrating on proper edge-setting techniques (Fig. 4.73B).

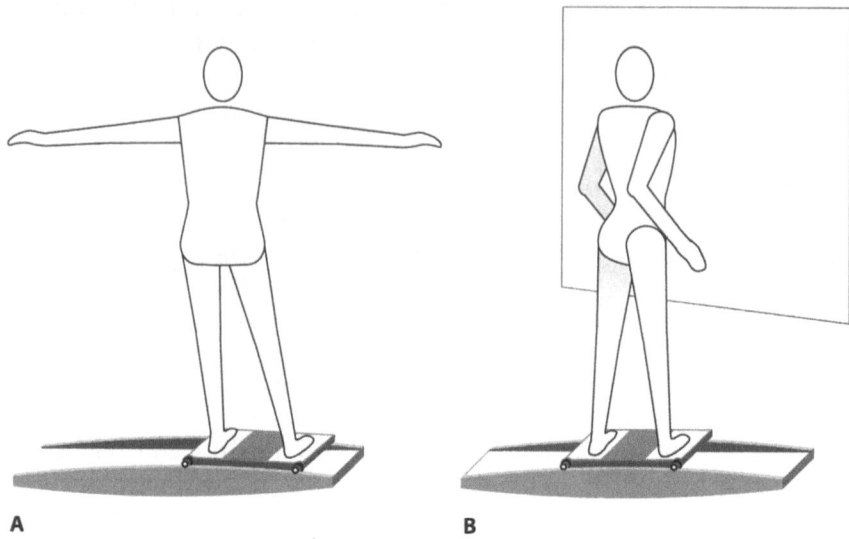

A   **B**

Fig. 4.73. Oscillations on the Skitter (**A**) with smooth weight changing; (**B**) as in slalom, fixating a mirror

Synergetics Phase

The patient performs the exercises of the cybernetics phase numbers 8, 9, 13, 15, 16 and 17 during simultaneous vestibular electrical stimulation placing the electrodes on the paravertebral muscles of the affected side and the opposite trapezius.

Home Protocol

The exercises have been subdivided according to the different phases of equilibrium, passing from supine to standing and to moving. In each phase, there is a progression from mechanics to synergetics exercises. They are not based on habituation mechanisms, but on sensorimotor learning phenomena.

Home exercises can never substitute for the therapeutic programs shown in the previous section, performed with the therapist. Home exercises complete the therapeutic period of treatment and maintain the obtained results.

A. Supine

1. With the legs flexed and feet on the bed rotate your pelvis rightward and leftward keeping your knees flexed and your legs together.

2. Lift your pelvis simultaneously extending your arms over your head. Then reposition your arms along the body lowering your pelvis.

3. Grasp a stick. Take your extended arms over your head and then return to the original position.

4. Rotate your head rightward and fixate a target on the lateral wall. Then straighten your head maintaining the visual fixation. Count up to 10 and then rotate your head.

5. Rotate your head leftward and fix a target on the lateral wall. Then straighten your head maintaining the visual fixation. Count up to 10 and then rotate your head.

6. From the supine position pass to the sitting position fixating a point straight in front of you.

7. From the supine position pass to the sitting position fixating a point sited on your right.

8. From the supine position pass to the sitting position fixating a point sited on your left.

B. Sitting

9. Move your head first slowly and then more rapidly in all directions fixating a target straight in front of you.

10. Look for three targets sited, respectively, in front of you, on your left and on your right. Fixate the front target, then move your head rapidly fixating the right-hand target. Now rotate your head leftward maintaining the fixation of the right-hand target. Fixate the frontal target. Now, suddenly, move your head leftward and fixate the left-hand target. Then rotate your head rightward maintaining the fixation of the left-hand target.

11. Inhale. Exhaling, bend forward holding your head on the right knee. Wait 10 s. Inhaling, return to the sitting position. Exhaling, bend forward holding your head on the left knee. Wait 10 s and then, inhaling, return to the sitting position.

12. Inhale. Exhaling, bend forward to pick up an object from the floor. Inhale and take it up over your head and then fixate it for 10 s. Inhale. Exhaling, bend forward and place the object back on the floor.

C. Standing

13. Hold a small object and then lift it over your head and fixate it. With your extended arms, move it in circles of increasing width maintaining the fixation of the object.

14. Repeat the exercise with eyes closed.

15. Repeat the exercise again standing on a soft mattress.

16. Hold a small object and lift it over your head. Fixate it. Inhale. Then exhale and bend yourself forward placing the object on the floor. Wait 10 s and then, inhaling, again lift the object over your head.
17. Hold a small object and lift it over your head. Fixate it. Lift it over your head and then, with your arms straight, move the object in circles of increasing width and, simultaneously bending your trunk and knees, place it on the floor.
18. Repeat the exercise on a soft mattress.

Dizziness and Vertigo Following Whiplash Injuries

Definitions of whiplash syndrome are controversial. Generally speaking, the syndrome includes symptoms following a traffic accident, usually a rear-end collision. These symptoms are varied and occur in various combinations:
- Orthopedic, such as neck pain and functional limitation of cervical movements.
- Neurological, such as paresthesias.
- Audiological, such as tinnitus and hypoacusia.
- Otorhinolaryngological, such as dysphagia and disphonias.
- Equilibriometric, such as vertigo and dizziness.
- Odontoiatric, such as disturbances of occlusions and temporo-mandibular joint pain.

Whiplash injury can be defined as a noncontact rapid (50 ms) acceleration-deceleration head-neck trauma. The different combinations of symptoms lead to the different syndromes described in the literature:
- Cervical syndrome.
- Traumatic cervical syndrome.
- Cervicocephalic syndrome.
- Cervicobrachial syndrome.

Whiplash injuries vary from minor to severe; generally the evolution of the whiplash is divide into three phases:
- The onset phase, involving local reactions with release of neuromediators, such as serotonin, histamine, bradykinin and classical inflammation.
- The recovery phase, locally characterized by synthesis of new collagenous fibers.
- The remodeling phase in which the neck or the body modify their positions and movement strategies in order to restore normal daily life activities.

During whiplash the kinematics of the cervical spine are completely disrupted. During the impact, the vertebrae do not reciprocally move harmonically such as during physiological antero- and retroflexion of the neck. Whiplash is characterized by transient, but not always temporary, reciprocal inversions of the different cervical segments. For example, in the last phase of anteroflexion there is an inversion in segments C1–C2 and C0–C1, while in the second phase of retroflexion an inversion of the segment C0–C1 is observed. The reciprocal inversions lead to ligament and soft tissue lesions, with a segmental dysregulation causing aspecific activation of nociceptive inputs and consequent somatomotor and sympathetic-motor dysfunctions. The nociceptive inputs, via interneurons and alpha-motoneurons, provoke a dysregulation of motoneurons for the flexors and extensors leading to asymmetrical hypertonus. Asymmetrical hypertonus is generally observed in trapezius and sternocleidomastoideus with consequent compression of the accessorius nerve, and in scalenii with compression of the brachial plexus, causing paresthesias. The dysregulation of the orthosympathetic cervical system causes activation of vasoconstrictive subsystems, not always localized to the involved segments. Vasoconstriction induces dystrophic impairment contributing to the cervicofacial and cervicobrachial symptoms.

Cervico and craniospinal injuries during acceleration-deceleration lead to head/neck proprioception disruption, causing transient and sometimes permanent abnormal proprioceptive information.

Whiplash is a true head trauma even without any contact of the head. Cerebral contusions or intracranial bleeding are extremely rare but abducens mono- and bilateral palsy and laryngeal palsy have been described. Neurovegetative symptoms and affective, cognitive symptoms are reported such as in postconcussion syndromes characterized by hyperesthesic-emotional and neuroasthenic syndrome including tinnitus, dysphasia, nausea, unsteadiness and vertigo. True neuropsychological disorders are frequent after whiplash.

The pathogenesis of otoneurological dysfunctions is still debated:
- Mechanical compression with dynamic stenosis of the vertebral arteria/ae.
- Sympathetic abnormal stimulation.
- Proprioceptive disorder especially from cervical and lumbar regions.
- Central vestibular system disorder.

Equilibrium impairment probably derives from different combinations of mechanisms. The kinematics of acceleration-deceleration is different, for example, for the driver, who usually resists the trauma by means of his or her arms on the wheel, and the passenger, who usually receives the impact forces completely and passively. Differences can be observed depending on whether the patient was wearing a safety belt during the impact: where a safety belt is worn the movement of the head and the neck is not sagittal but torsional, with torsion having the first dorsal vertebrae as the fulcrum. The direction of the torsional component is different: counterclockwise for the passenger, clockwise in the driver. Furthermore, the impact is rarely caused by a perfect sagittal rear-end collision, while the impact very often causes a rotational acceleration of the car. Torsional and angular acceleration cause brain microlesions in different parts, and this can lead to different combinations of signs and symptoms in the so-called whiplash syndrome.

Following whiplash, either with mechanical lesions on cervical dynamics or with central dysfunctions, some modifications of patient posture are usually observed: the head modifies its position with antalgic flexion, thereby reducing its rotational and lateroflexion movements; during normal movements, rotation of the body is along the trunk and not the neck; with whiplash the trunk is ipsilaterally rotated with respect to the side of lesion, the pelvis is rotated according to the head's antalgic position, and the position of center of gravity (CoG) is modified.

In the months following the trauma, the erector paravertebral muscles become hypotonic and the prevalence of flexors induces a forward displacement of the CoG facilitating forward falling. Rotation of the trunk increases unsteadiness and forward CoG displacement provokes a relative flexion of the legs to resist the falling and dearrangement of the normal combination of ankle and hip strategies. In fact the Equitest shows a prevalence of ankle strategy and delayed motor control test latencies in both backward and forward translations.

From a cybernetics point of view, equilibrium disorders are provoked by distortion and desynchronization of the proprioceptive chain:
- Modification of the proprioceptive cervical inputs to the vestibular nuclei and reticular formation.
- Desynchronization between special vestibular inputs and general cervical inputs regarding head position and movement.
- Modification of the cervicospinal reflexes.

Treatment must aim to:
1. Restore cervicodorsal mobility.
2. Restore dorsolumbar mobility.

3. Reorganize proprioceptive information from the neck and the pelvis.
4. Avoid secondary damage characterized by a reduction of the movement of the body along the neck with involvement of the thoracolumbar segment and pelvis.
5. Restore head-neck coordination.
6. Restore the control of head stabilization during gait.
7. Reorganize the self-perception of posture.

Because, as we saw above, whiplash injuries cause different and variable damage and symptoms, the following protocol is only a general guide about what action is useful in a patient after such a trauma. In every patient suffering vertigo and dizziness, but especially in this case of vertigo and dizziness, treatment closely tailored to the patient is necessary. The following protocol is for the treatment of vertigo and dizziness, but it is obvious that it is very often also necessary to conduct physiotherapy of the cervical and thoracic spine with soft mobilization and relaxation massage.

Exercises in the Gymnasium

Mechanics Phase
1. The patient holds his two knees to the chest, simultaneously helping, gently, with the hands (Fig. 4.74).
2. With the legs flexed and the feet on the bed, the patient rotates his pelvis rightward and leftward keeping his knees flexed and legs together (Fig. 4.75).
3. The patient lifts his pelvis simultaneously extending his arms over his head. He then repositions his arms along the body lowering his pelvis (Fig. 4.76).
4. In the quadrupedal position the patient simultaneously extends the right arm and the left leg and then repeats the exercise with the left arm and the right leg (Fig. 4.77).
5. In the prone position the patient lifts his left arm and right leg, holding his forehead over the bed. He then repeats with the right arm and the left leg (Fig. 4.78).
6. The patient repeats the exercise as above but simultaneously also lifting the head.
7. The patient inhales. Exhaling, he bends forward holding his head on the right knee. He waits 10 s. Inhaling, he returns to the sitting position. Exhaling, he bends forward taking his head on the left knee. He waits 10 s and then inhaling he returns to the sitting position (Figs. 4.79, 4.80).

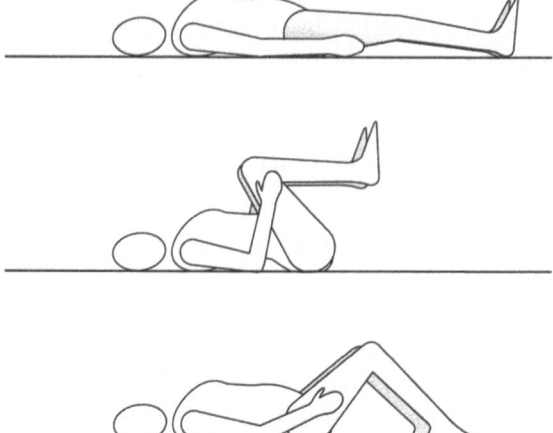

Fig. 4.74. Patient holds both knees against the chest

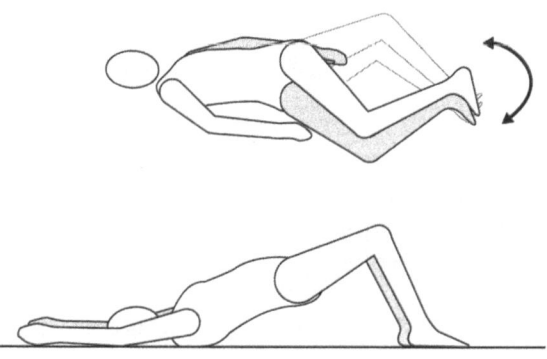

Fig. 4.75. Rotation of the pelvis

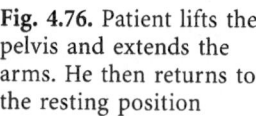

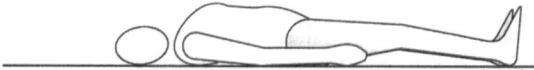

Fig. 4.76. Patient lifts the pelvis and extends the arms. He then returns to the resting position

Fig. 4.77. Alternating extension of one arm and the opposite leg

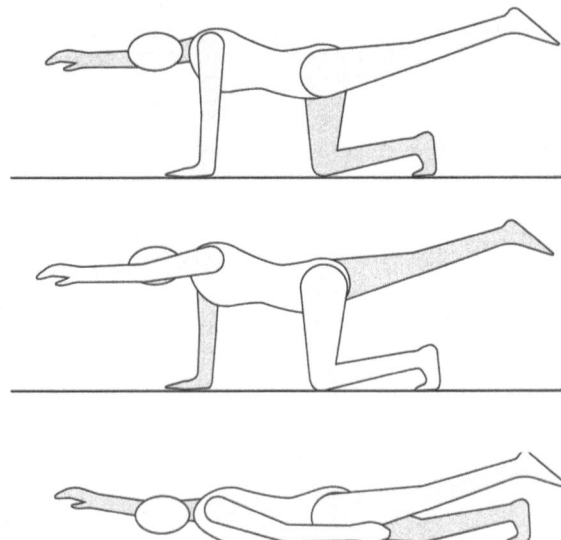

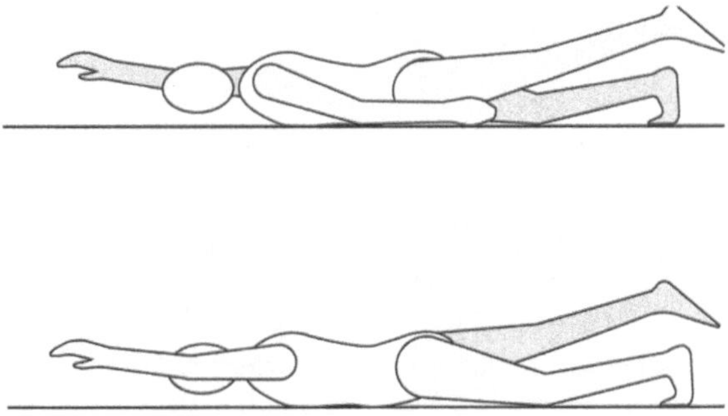

Fig. 4.78. In the prone position simultaneous extension of one arm and the opposite leg

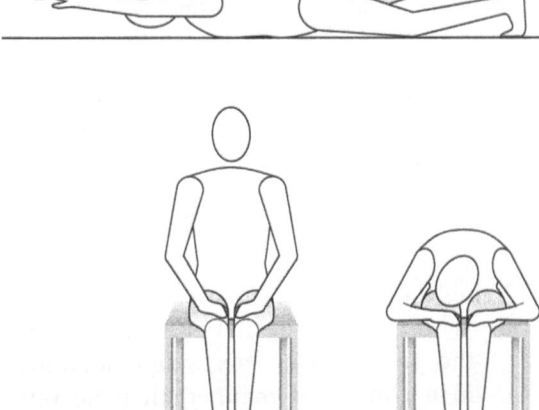

Fig. 4.79. Bending the trunk

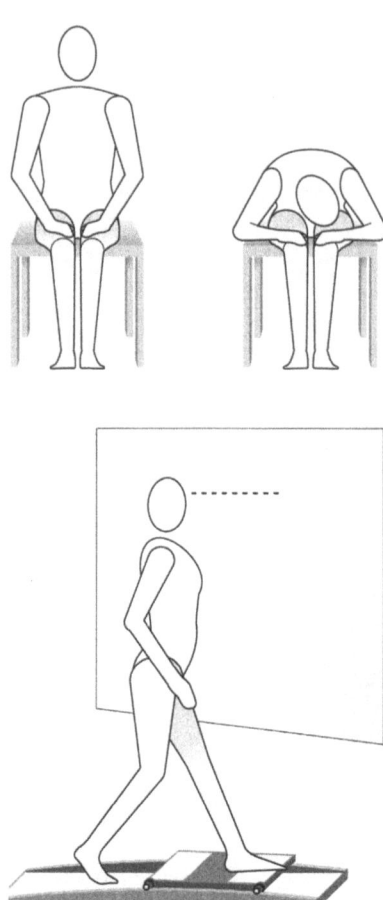

Fig. 4.80. Bending the trunk

Fig. 4.81. Extension of the forward leg

8. Using the Skitter
   a) With one foot on the end cap and the other across the footpad, the patient keeps his weight forward and extends the front leg in a controlled manner, then he returns slowly to the starting position and repeats the exercise (Fig. 4.81).
   b) With one foot on the end cap and the other across the footpad, the patient keeps his weight backward and extends the rear leg in a controlled manner, then returning slowly to the starting position and repeating the exercise (Fig. 4.82).
   c) The patient maintains equilibrium on one leg with the other extended or flexed or with one leg lateral. The therapist helps the patient to maintain equilibrium and to correct his posture. A

Fig. 4.82. Backward leg
extension

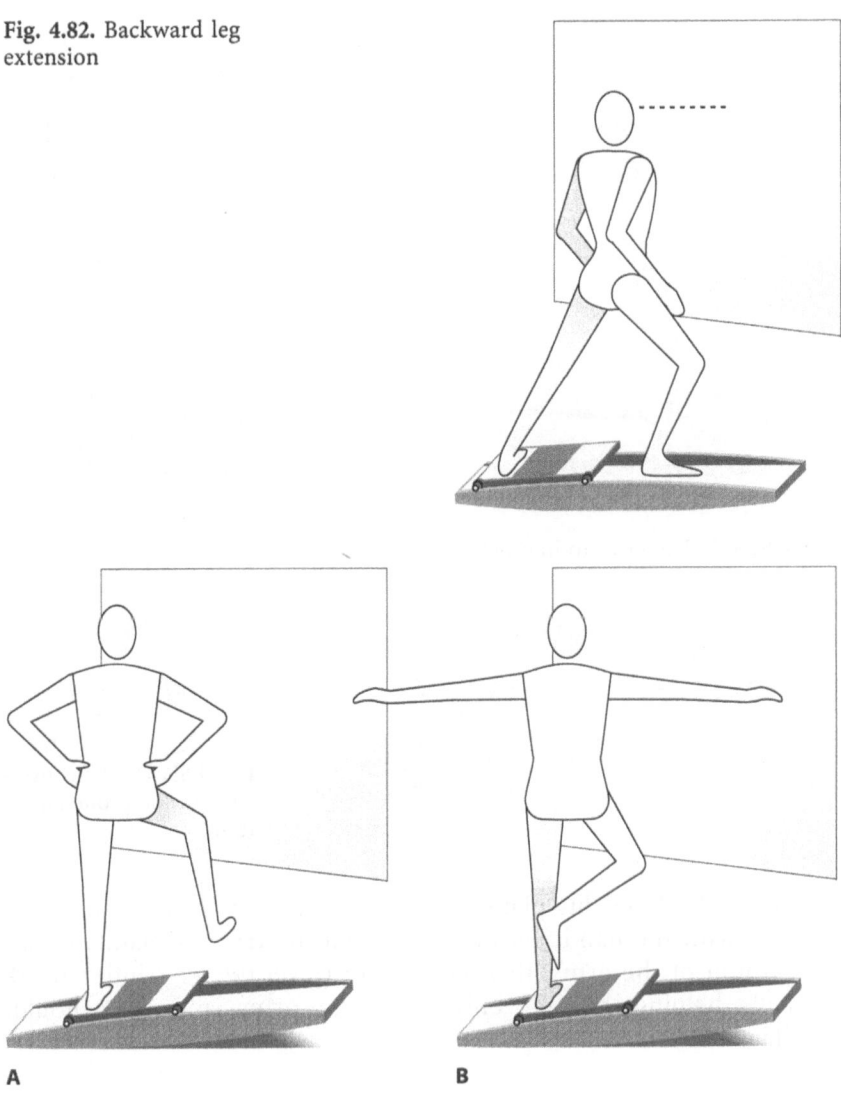

Fig. 4.83A, B. Equilibrium on one leg

mirror facilitates the correction of the postural equilibrium
strategy (Fig. 4.83A, B).

d) The patient keeps the knees straight pushing the skate forward
with the toes and pulling back with the heels. He has to concentrate on using only the ankles and calves, while all the other
muscles are relaxed (Fig. 4.84).

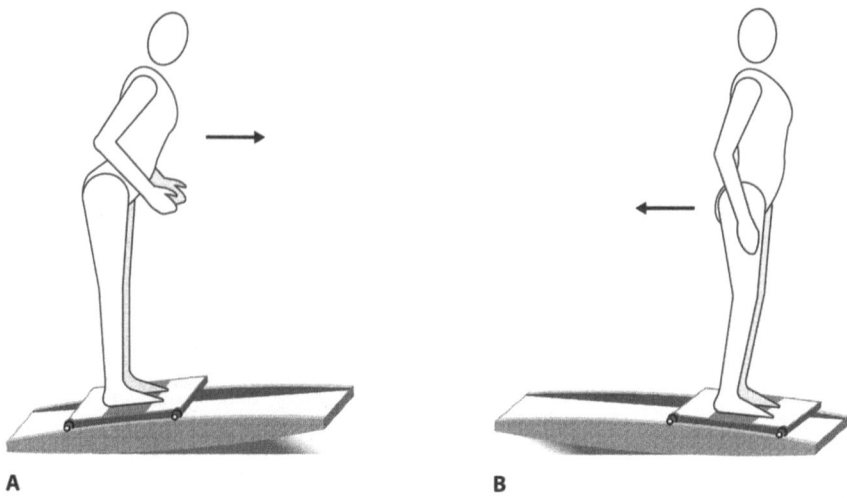

A   **B**

Fig. 4.84 A, B. Exercises to improve ankle stability

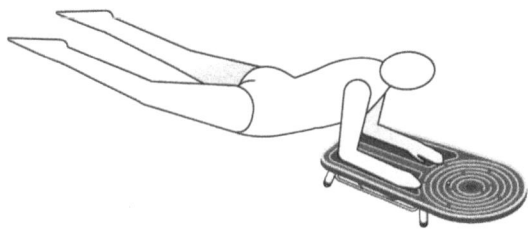

Fig. 4.85. Daedalus exercises in the prone position

9. Using the Daedalus platform: the patient starts in the prone position with the hands on the table. First, he tries to maintain equilibrium of the arms, then he tries to travel the labyrinth with the ball, helping himself only with the arms and the shoulder (Fig. 4.85).

Cybernetics Phase

10. The patient fixates a target on the ceiling and slowly moves his head rightward and leftward.
11. The patient looks for two equidistant targets on the ceiling and then he fixates them alternately first moving only the eyes and then moving only the head.
12. The patient in the supine position moves to the sitting position fixating a point straight in front of him (Fig. 4.86).
13. From the supine position the patient moves to the sitting position fixating a point on his right.

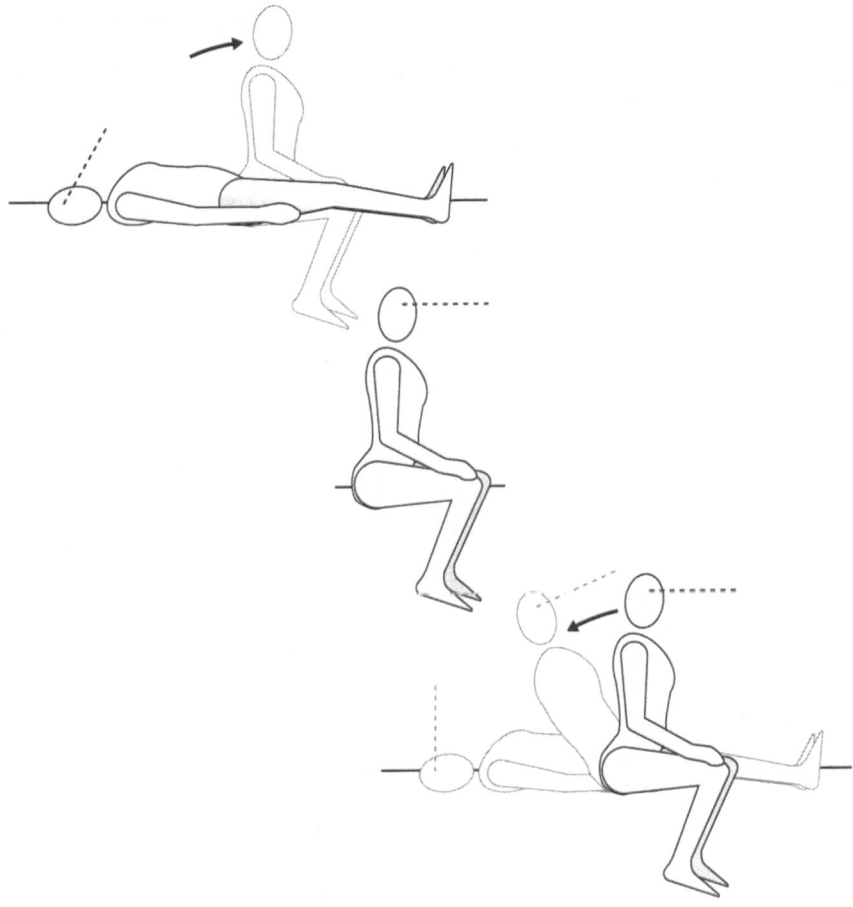

Fig. 4.86. From the supine to the sitting position and vice versa

14. From the supine position the patient moves to the sitting position fixating a point on his left.
15. The patient moves up and down a step, fixating a target according to the following sequence:
    Right foot up left foot up right foot down
    Left foot down left foot up right foot up
    Left foot down right foot down

He then repeats the exercise with the eyes closed.
16. Using the Rettiks.
    a) The patient moves his head first slowly and then faster in all directions fixating a target straight in front of him (Fig. 4.87).

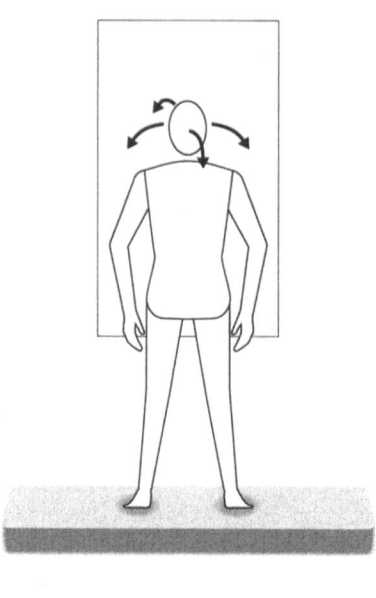

Fig. 4.87. Movements of the head in all directions standing on the mattress

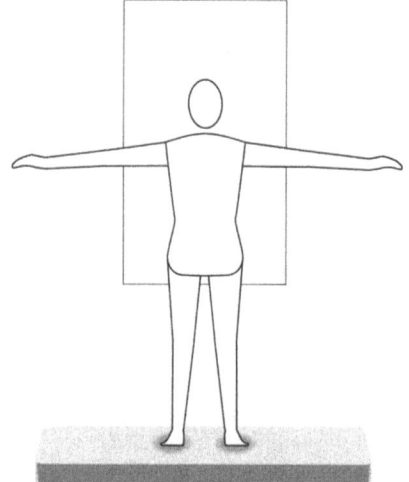

Fig. 4.88. Correct alignment of posture standing on the mattress

b) The patient fixates himself in a mirror and aligns his position correctly. He then maintains equilibrium for 1 min and then closes his eyes visualizing his correct position while remaining still in the same position for at least 1 min (Fig. 4.88).

c) The patient fixates himself in a mirror. He then oscillates to and fro and from side to side, around his ankles keeping his pelvis still (ankle strategy) (Fig. 4.89).

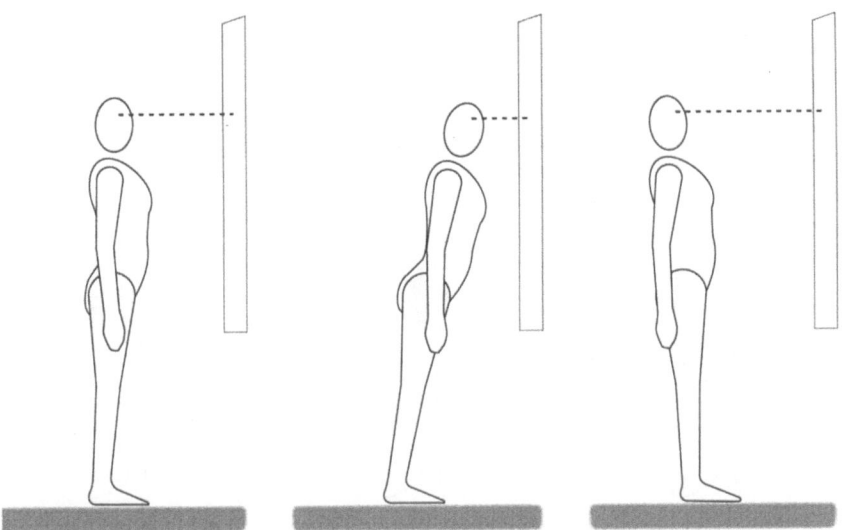

Fig. 4.89. Ankle oscillations

    d) The patient fixates himself in a mirror; keeping his feet still he bends the trunk to and fro and from side to side (hip strategy) (Fig. 4.90).

    e) The patient holds a small object and lifts it over his head while fixating it. He lifts it over his head and then, with arms straight, he moves the object in circles of increasing width (Fig. 4.91); then, simultaneously bending his trunk and his knees, he places it on the floor (Fig. 4.92).

    f) The patient performs steps fixating a target in front of him (Fig. 4.93).

    g) In the quadrupedal position on a double mattress, the patient performs synchronization exercises of the arm and leg (Fig. 4.94).

16. Using the Skitter.

    a) The patient steps on footpads with the feet centrally positioned. He then concentrates on a proper posture using a mirror to look at his reflection and begins to transfer his weight from one foot to the other with a smooth flowing motion (Fig. 4.95A).

    b) The therapist destabilizes the skate and the patient maintains equilibrium and rhythmic changing of the weight (Fig. 4.95B).

    c) The patient moves his weight rhythmically and slowly. As his rhythms increase he moves closer to the bumpers at each end,

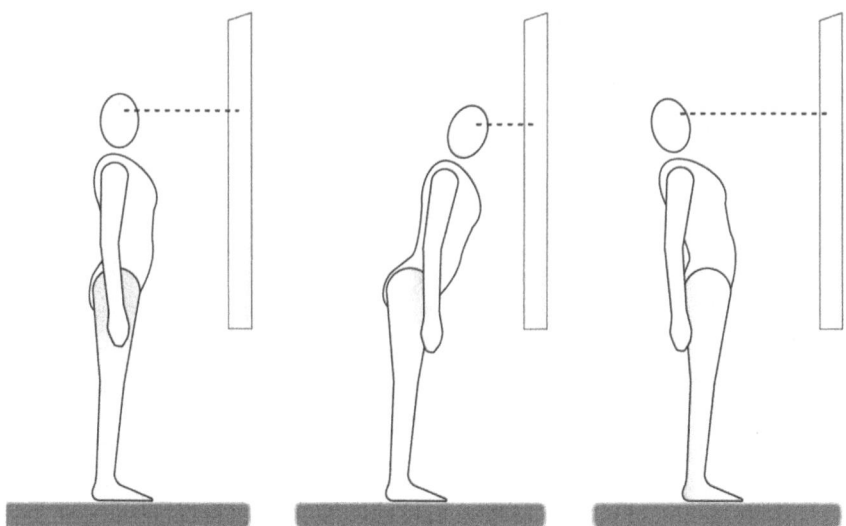

Fig. 4.90. Hip oscillations

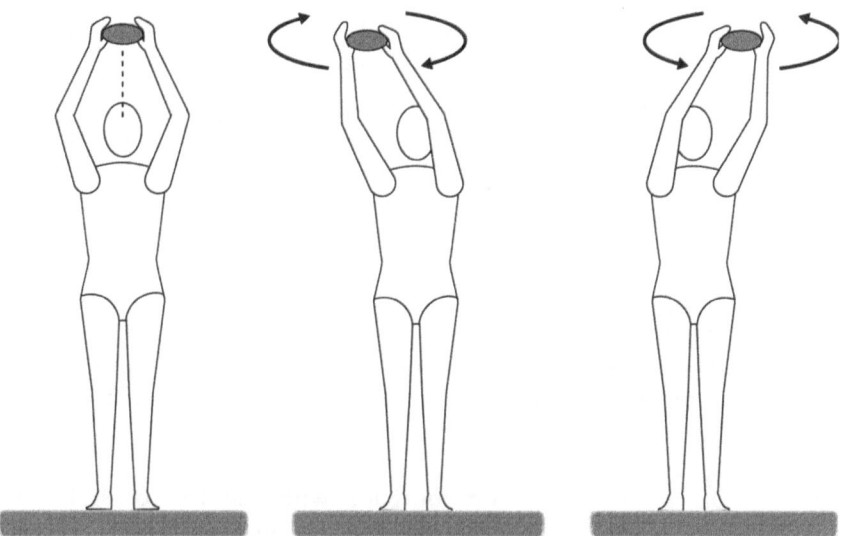

Fig. 4.91. Circular movements of a small object over the head

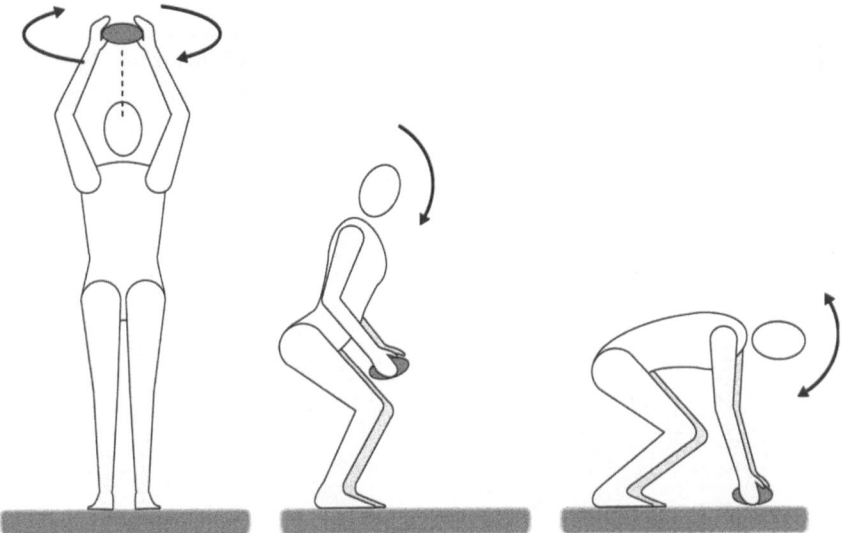

Fig. 4.92. Circular movements of a small object, bending the trunk and placing the object on the floor

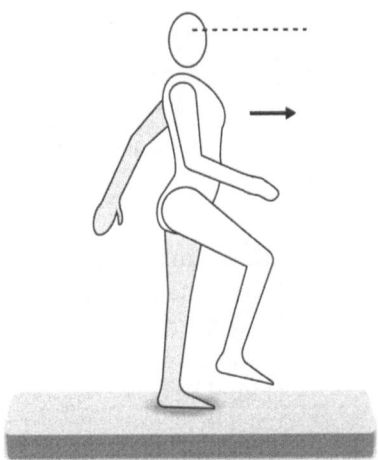

Fig. 4.93. Stepping on the mattress

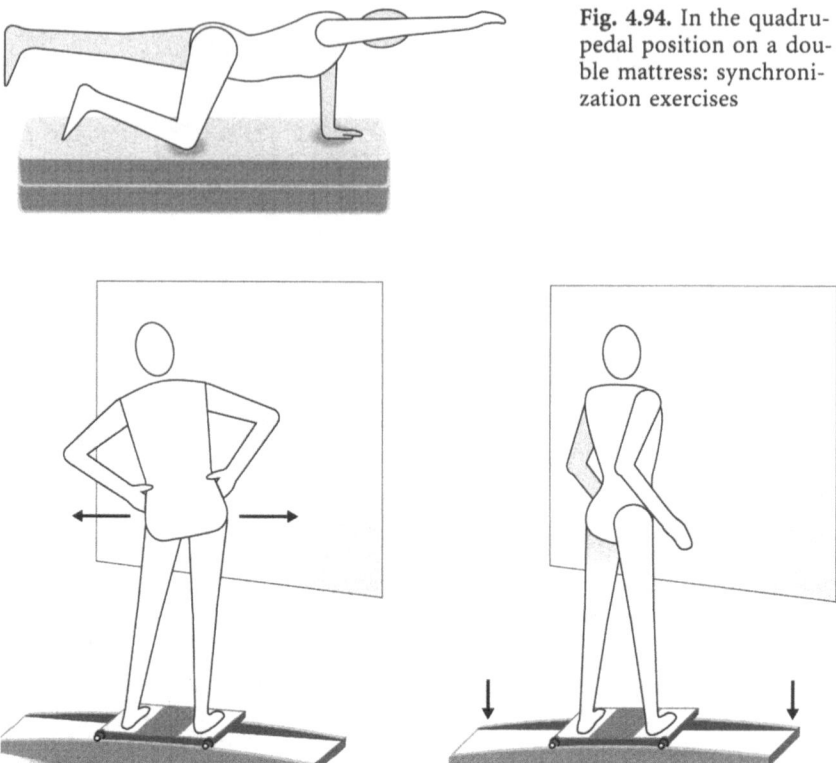

Fig. 4.94. In the quadrupedal position on a double mattress: synchronization exercises

Fig. 4.95. Patient changes weight on the Skitter (**A**) and the therapist destabilizes the skate (**B**)

always maintaining a good upright posture with eyes focused in the mirror and paying attention to his balance. The exercise is performed with limited upper body movement as in slalom without including upper body motion, as in giant slalom (Fig. 4.96).

Synergetics Phase

17. The patient extends his right arm and lifts his thumb. Then he slowly moves his arm to and fro first in a horizontal direction and then in a vertical direction. He follows his thumb with eyes only, first slowly and then increasing progressively the velocity of thumb displacement.

18. As above but simultaneously moving also the head while trying to maintain the eyes still.

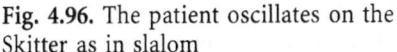

Fig. 4.96. The patient oscillates on the Skitter as in slalom

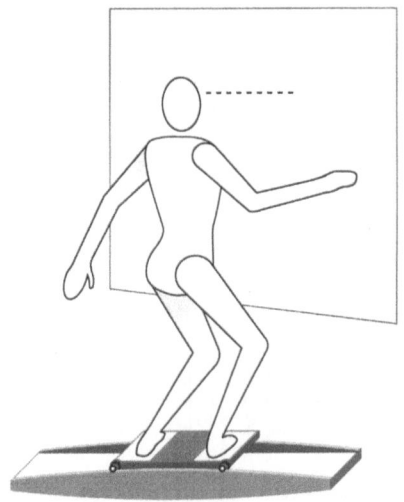

19. The patient opens a book in front of him. Then he moves it away from him by extending his arms while reading it at the same time. He then moves it closer to him slowly, trying to read it, then moves it away again and he repeats the exercise several times.

20. Using the Rettiks
    a) The patient stands on the mattress and then he moves up and down a step, moving his head to and fro, during fixation of a target placed on a mirror, according to the following sequence:
    Right foot up left foot up right foot down
    Left foot down left foot up right foot up
    Left foot down right foot down
    b) The patient opens a book in front of him and reads it, simultaneously moving it to and fro and right and left.
    c) The patient opens a book in front of him, then moves it away from him extending his arms while reading it. Then he moves it closer to him slowly, trying to read it. He then repeats the exercise several times.

21. Using the Skitter: the patient stands in a comfortable and stable position on the footpads. With his thumbs and limbs extended he tries to touch visual targets placed in different positions on a facing mirror (Fig. 4.97) according to the commands of the therapist.

22. Using the Daedalus
    a) The patient stands on the table, with the feet parallel, grasping the sticks placed in the anterior holes and maneuvers the ball through the labyrinth (Fig. 4.98).

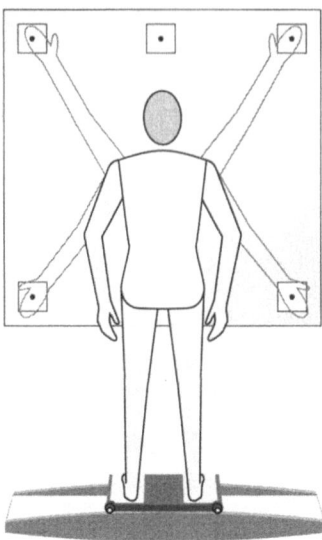

Fig. 4.97. Standing on the Skitter the patient touches different targets placed on a mirror

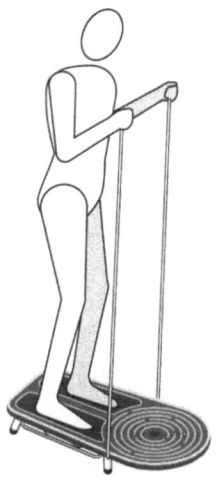

Fig. 4.98. The patient maneuvers the ball through the labyrinth grasping the sticks placed in the anterior holes

b) The patient stands on the table with the left foot placed anteriorly while the left stick is in a posterior position, like the position of a step. He maneuvers the ball through the labyrinth. Then the positions of the feet and the sticks are reversed (Fig. 4.99).

Fig. 4.99. The patient maneuvers the ball through the labyrinth with the left foot and right stick forward and the opposite side backward, as during gait

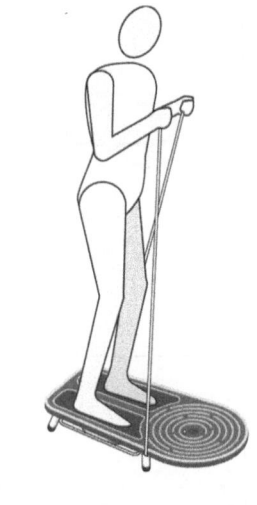

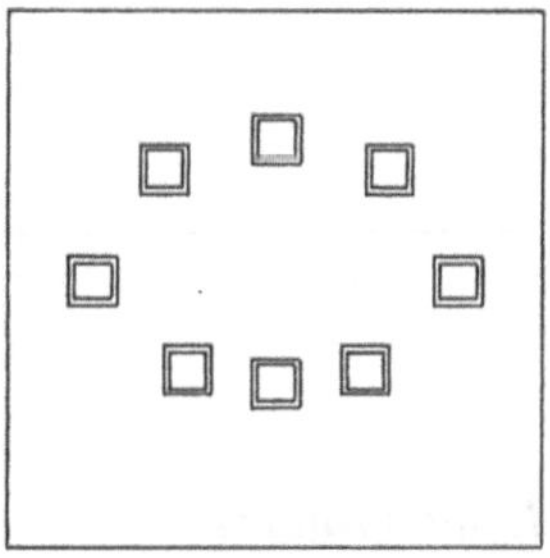

Fig. 4.100. Example of target position to improve ankle strategy (Balance Master, reproduced by courtesy of NeuroCom International, Inc., Clackamas, Oregon, USA)

23. By visual feedback devices
   a) The position of the target is generally that which reproduces the perimeter of the limits of stability. To improve ankle strategy the target is placed in a large circle with a slow rhythm of target displacement, while to improve hip strategy the target is placed in a smaller circle (Fig. 4.100), with a fast pacing. According to the previous evaluation of the patient, the target may placed especially in the anterior, posterior or lateral positions.
   b) The same exercises can be performed with the patient wearing visual prisms inducing a slight convergence (2–3°) with the bases of both prisms placed outward.
   c) The targets are positioned in order to improve the laterolateral oscillation strategy. Also in this case the exercises can be performed with the patient wearing prisms (Figs. 4.101, 4.102).

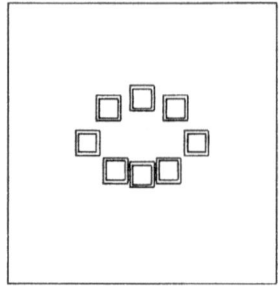

Fig. 4.101. Example of target position to improve hip strategy (Balance Master, reproduced by courtesy of NeuroCom International, Inc, Clackamas, Oregon, USA)

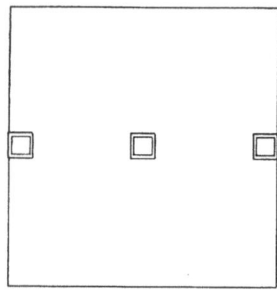

Fig. 4.102. Example of target position to improve lateral sway (Balance Master, reproduced by courtesy of NeuroCom International, Inc., Clackamas, Oregon, USA)

Home Protocol

The exercises are subdivided according to the different phases of equilibrium, from supine to standing to moving. In each phase, there is a progression from mechanics to synergetics exercises.

Home exercises can never substitute for the therapeutic programs shown in the previous section performed with the therapist. Home exercises complete the therapy and maintain the results obtained.

A. Supine
1. Hold your two knees to the chest, simultaneously helping, gently, with the hands.
2. Put a pillow under your leg. Bind a 2-kg weight to your ankle with the flexed knee, then extend it alternating the right and left legs.
3. With the flexed legs and the feet on the bed rotate your pelvis rightward and leftward keeping your knees flexed and your legs together.
4. Lift your pelvis simultaneously extending your arms over your head. Then reposition your arms along the body lowering your pelvis.

5. Fixate a target on the ceiling and slowly move your head rightward and leftward.

6. Look for two equidistant targets on the ceiling and then fixate them alternately first moving only the eyes and then moving only the head.

7. In the quadrupedal position, inhale and arch your back (hyperkyphosis) holding your head between your arms. Then exhale bending your head and rotating the pelvis in hyperlordosis.

8. From the supine position move to the sitting position fixating a target straight in front of you.

9. In the quadrupedal position simultaneously extend the right arm and the left leg. Then repeat with the left arm and the right leg.

10. In the prone position lift your left arm and right leg simultaneously also lifting the head. Then repeat with the right arm and the left leg.

B. Sitting

11. Extend your right arm and lift your thumb. Move your arm slowly to and fro first in a horizontal direction and then in a vertical direction. Pursue your thumb with the eyes only, first slowly and then increasing progressively the velocity of thumb displacement.

12. As above but simultaneously moving also the head while trying to maintain the eyes still.

13. Move your head first slowly and then faster in all directions fixating a target straight in front of you.

14. Inhale. Exhaling, bend forward holding your head on the right knee. Wait 10 s. Inhaling, return to the sitting position. Exhaling, bend forward holding your head on the left knee. Wait 10 s and then inhale and return to the sitting position.

15. Inhale. Exhaling, bend forward to pick up an object from the floor. Inhale and take it up over your head and then fixate it for 10 s. Inhale. Exhaling, bend forward and place the object on the floor.

16. Open a book in front of you. Read it while at the same time moving the book right and left and then to and fro.

C. Standing

17. Fixate yourself in a mirror. Align your position correctly. Maintain equilibrium for 1 min and then close your eyes visualizing your correct position and remain in this position for at least 1 min.

18. Repeat the same exercise, standing on a soft mattress.

19. Fixate yourself in a mirror; then, keeping your feet still, bend your trunk to and fro and right and left with eyes closed while standing on a soft mattress.

20. Hold a small object and lift it over your head. Fixate it. Inhale. Then exhale and bend yourself forward placing the object on the floor. Wait 10 s and then inhaling again lift the object over your head.
21. Standing on a soft mattress, hold a small object and lift it over your head. Fixate it. Lift it over your head and then, with your arms straight, move the object in circles of increasing width and, simultaneously bending your trunk and knees, place it on the floor.
D. Moving
22. Stepping with eyes closed, moving the head to and fro.
23. Stepping while reading a book.
24. Stepping on a soft mattress, reading a book.
25. Go up and down a step, moving your head to and fro, according to the following sequence:
Right foot up left foot up right foot down
Left foot down left foot up right foot up
Left foot down right foot down

Dizziness in the Elderly

Dizziness and unsteadiness are frequent symptoms with aging. They are particularly important because they decrease the social autonomy of aged subjects and they are often the cause of falls. The causes of dizziness are always multifactorial. There is evidence that aging affects multiple sensory inputs, as well as the ability of the musculoskeletal system and central nervous system to perform sensorimotor integration. The elderly are characterized by perturbation at several levels, including the motor and sensory levels (decreases in muscle mass, increases in the threshold of vibratory sensations) and the cognitive level (memory processes, attention span). Gait instability, especially in older women, may be compromised by the combination of increased body weight and decreased muscle strength.

Somatosensation is the primary sense that triggers the automatic postural responses when a standing adult experiences a sudden horizontal support surface displacement. The activation of the distal leg muscles has short latency and it may serve as the primary defense mechanism, with the supplement of visual and vestibular inputs, to prevent falls when a person encounters an unexpected support surface displacement, such as a slip. With advancing age the thresholds of joint position sense, vibration sense and cutaneous sense increase. Older subjects show a higher threshold for detecting movement in the metatarsophalangeal joint.

Reduced peripheral proprioceptive information in the elderly probably plays an important role. There is a close relationship between increased sway and impaired vibration sense in the legs. Cutaneous and proprioceptive sensation thresholds increase with age. The importance of cervical proprioception is stressed by some authors. Alterations that develop as a result of the gradual loss of function of the receptors is considered an inevitable concomitant of the aging process. Abnormalities in the reflexogenic functions of the cervical articular mechanoreceptors make a significant contribution to the disorders of posture and gait that afflict old people.

Reduced visual acuity is frequent with age. It appears to be accompanied by increased postural sway, particularly in the anteroposterior direction. The following deficits in focal vision have been found in the older adult: decreased visual acuity, restriction of visual field, poor depth perception, and losses in contrast sensitivity at the intermediate and high spatial frequencies. It is thus hypothesized that a decline in balance control abilities in older adults may be partially attributable to these functional decrements in focal vision.

Older adults show diminished sensitivity to a moving target with low spatial frequencies, especially when this target moves at a high speed. Older adults not only have difficulty in perceiving a moving object, but also have difficulty in perceiving self-motion with reference to the external space. In older fallers also the perception of verticality and horizontality is impaired compared to older nonfallers.

While the vestibular system plays an important role in resolving sensory conflicts that can be introduced by moving external space or surface, the number of vestibular hair cells has been reported to be reduced by 20%–40% in healthy adults 70 years and older when compared to young adults and the number of vestibular nerve fibers has also been found to decrease with age. Changes in the vestibular reflexes have also been described. In this way the caloric nystagmus is influenced by age and the threshold for rotatory nystagmus is increased, the postrotation reaction is changed, and nystagmus frequency increases together with a reduction of the amplitude.

In older patients a more frequent presence of central components or of a central pathology is expected such as typical neurological diseases, the influence of vertebrobasilar insufficiency and cardiovascular and degenerative changes in the CNS. A disturbance in the integrating mechanisms in the brainstem and cerebellum is common as a result of ischemia. Cerebrovascular disease may often have resulted in preexisting central nervous disease, and compensation of vestibular injuries is fragile and may break down if there is subsequent additional damage to any of the mechanisms responsible.

In conclusion, dizziness in the elderly is typically caused by multiple deficits, multiple deficits that can add up to produce disability disproportionate to their individual contributions.

Rehabilitation is an important step in the treatment of vertigo and dizziness in the elderly, but it usually needs to be achieved with modifications of lifestyle, home environment and pharmacotherapy. Sedative drugs are best generally avoided while drugs improving cognitive and motor skills are preferred.

Rehabilitative treatment aims to:
1. Improve ankle, hip and neck mobility.
2. Increase antigravitational muscle tone.
3. Improve balance reactions.
4. Ameliorate motor coordination.
5. Improve attention to balance phenomena.
6. Correct the internal representation of posture.

Each aged subject presents an individual picture of multiple sensorimotor involvement, some with greater involvement of the sensorial aspects, some with greater involvement of the motor aspects and some with greater involvement of the cognitive aspects. Thus the treatment protocol needs to be strictly personalized, adapting each phase to each patient. In some subjects attention must be paid to the mechanics phase (motor involvement), in some the cybernetics phase will need particular attention (sensorimotor involvement) while in others the synergetics phase will provide the key for treatment (cognitive-motor involvement).

Exercises in the Gymnasium

Mechanics Phase
1. The patient holds his left knee against the chest, then extends his leg and holds his right knee against the chest. When he holds the knee against the chest, he applies gentle traction to the flexed leg with the hands (Fig. 4.103A).
2. The patient holds both knees against the chest, simultaneously helping with the hands (Fig. 4.103B).
3. The patient extends his left arm over his head and simultaneously holds the right flexed leg to the chest, helping with his hand. He maintains this position for 10 s and then repeats the exercise with the opposite arm and leg (Fig. 4.104).

Fig. 4.103A, B. Flexions of the knees

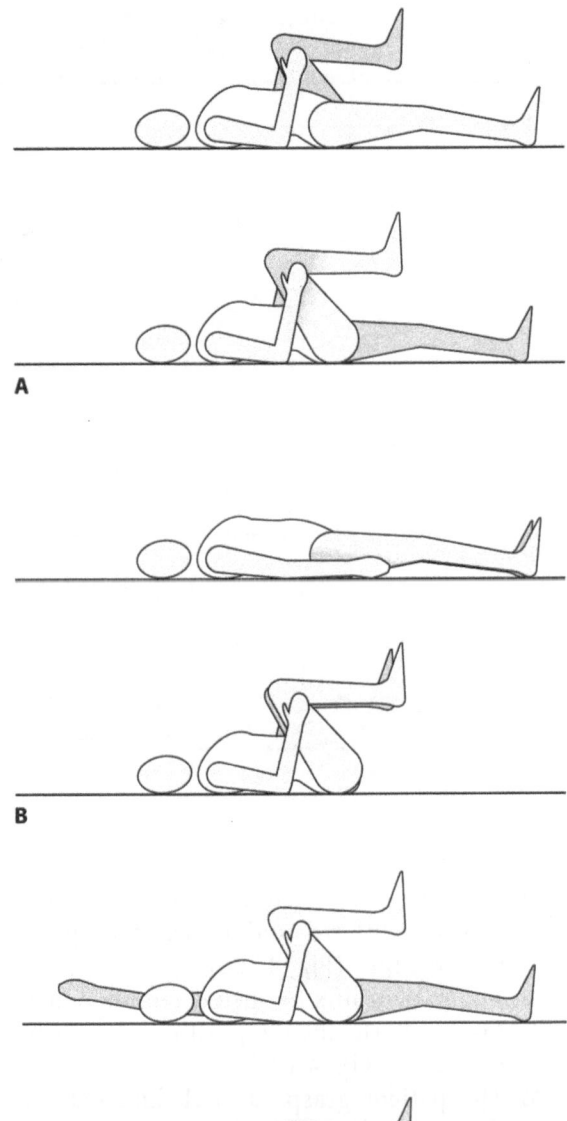

A

B

Fig. 4.104. Flexion of the knee and extension of the opposite arm

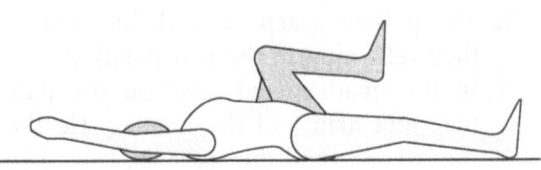

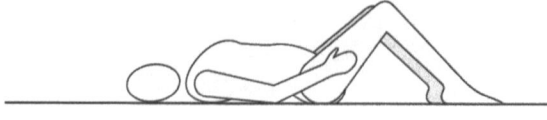

Fig. 4.105. Rotation of the pelvis

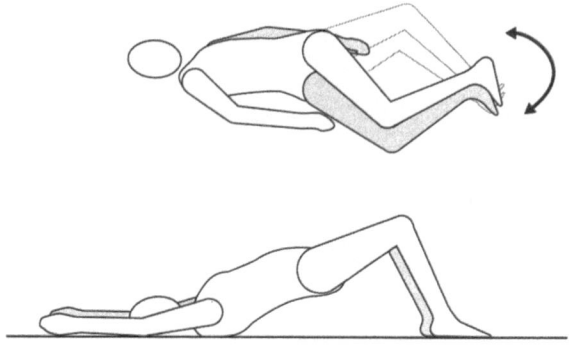

Fig. 4.106. Lifting the pelvis

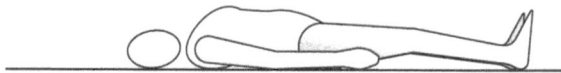

4. With the legs flexed and the feet on the bed the patient rotates his pelvis rightward and leftward keeping his knees flexed and his legs together (Fig. 4.105).
5. The patient lifts his pelvis simultaneously extending his arms over his head. He then repositions his arms along the body lowering his pelvis (Fig. 4.106).
6. The patient grasps a stick and extends his arms over his head, then returning to the rest position.
7. In the quadrupedal position the patient simultaneously extends the right arm and the left leg. He then repeats the exercise with the left arm and the right leg (Fig. 4.107).
8. In the quadrupedal position the patient arches his back for hyperkyphosis of the thoracolumbar spine (Fig. 4.108).
9. The patient moves his head, first slowly and then more rapidly, in all directions, fixating a target straight in front of him.

Fig. 4.107. Synchronization of arm-leg extension

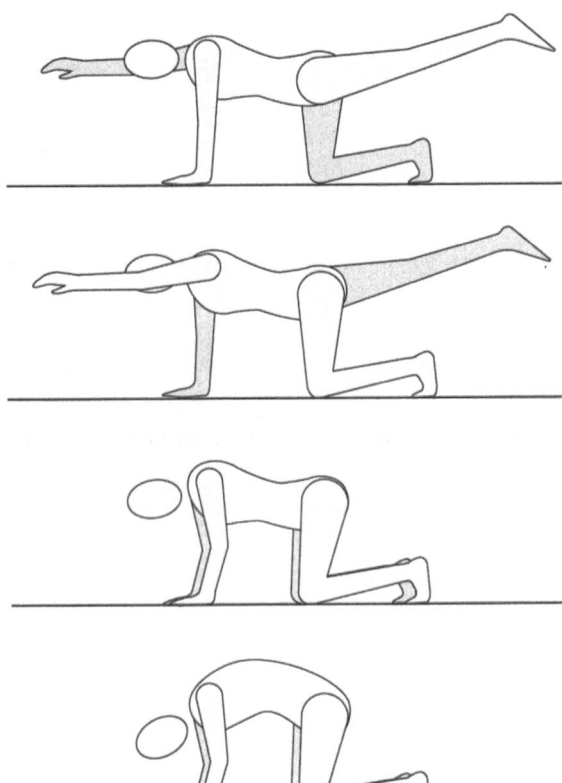

Fig. 4.108. In the quadrupedal position the patient arches the trunk

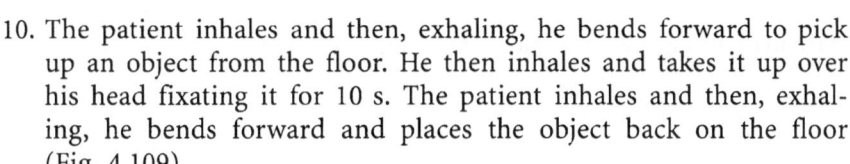

10. The patient inhales and then, exhaling, he bends forward to pick up an object from the floor. He then inhales and takes it up over his head fixating it for 10 s. The patient inhales and then, exhaling, he bends forward and places the object back on the floor (Fig. 4.109).
11. With the hands on a chair the patient lifts himself on his tiptoes and maintains this position for 30 s (Fig. 4.110A).
12. With the hands on a table the patient lifts himself on his heels and maintains this position for 30 s (Fig. 4.110B).
13. The patient performs steps on the floor with the eyes open (Fig. 4.111).
14. Using the Skitter: the patient holds his knees straight pushing the skate forward with the toes and pulling it back with the heels. He needs to concentrate on using only the ankles and calves, keeping all the other muscles relaxed (Fig. 4.112).

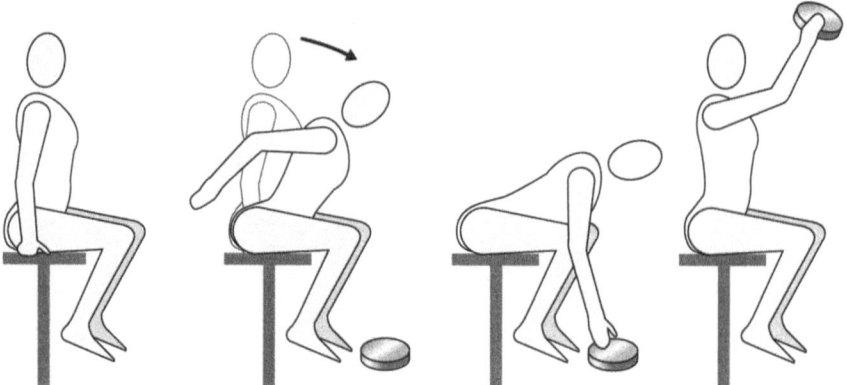

Fig. 4.109. Picking up and lifting an object from the floor

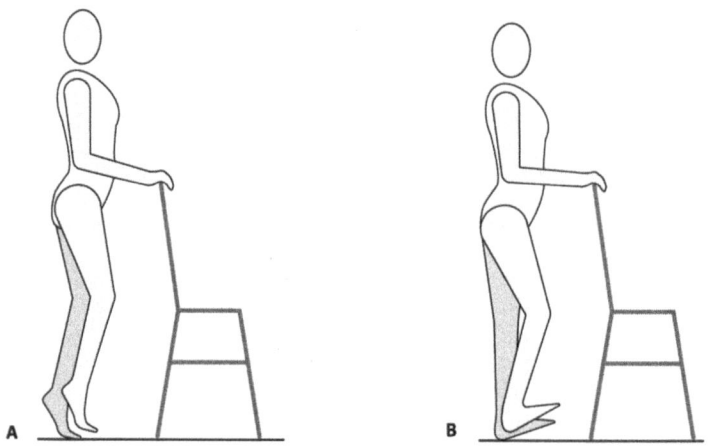

Fig. 4.110. Rising onto the tiptoes (**A**) and the heels (**B**)

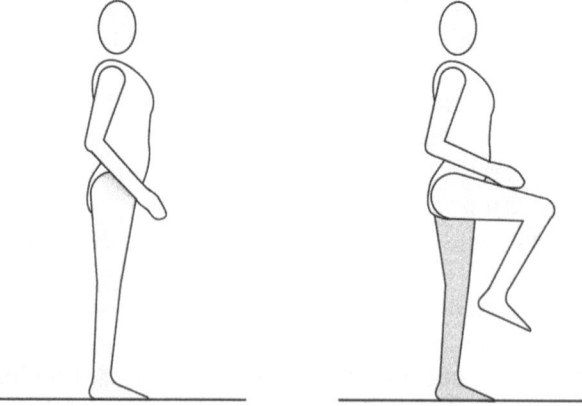

Fig. 4.111. Stepping

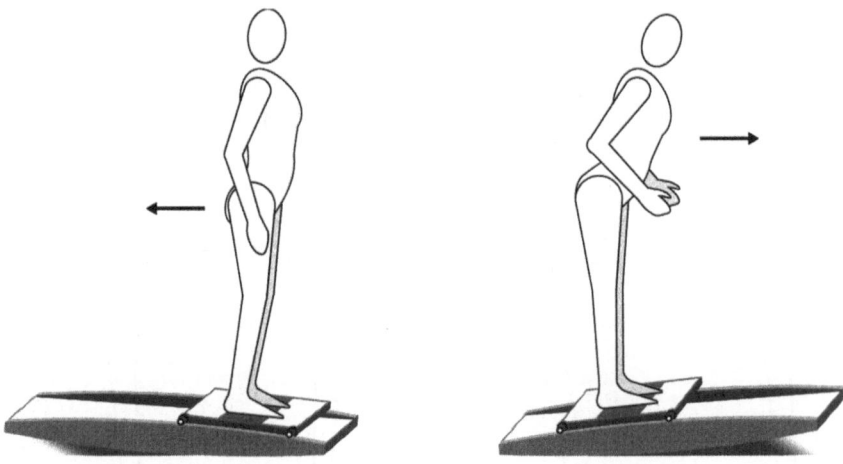

Fig. 4.112. Ankle stability exercises

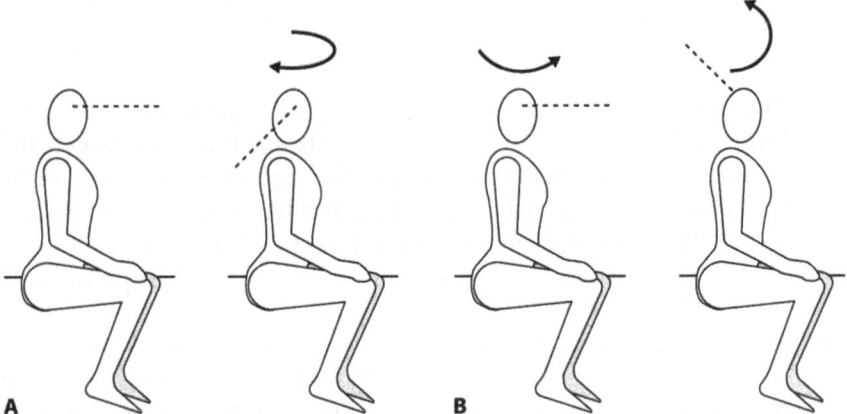

Fig. 4.113A, B. Turning the head fixating a target

Cybernetics Phase

15. The patient turns his head rightward and fixates a target on the lateral wall. Then he straightens his head maintaining the visual fixation and counting up to 10; then he turns his head (Fig. 4.113A).

16. The patients turns his head leftward and fixates a target on the lateral wall. He then straightens his head, maintaining the visual fixation and counting up to 10, then turning his head (Fig. 4.113B).

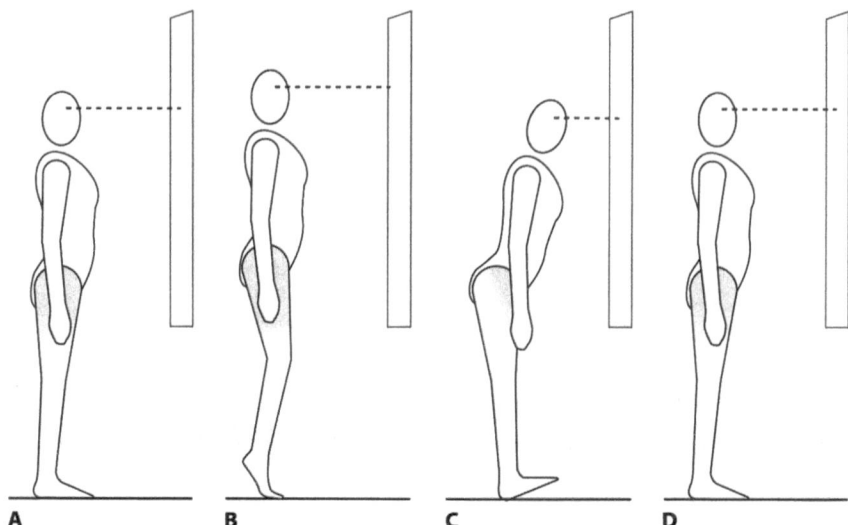

Fig. 4.114. Correct alignment in front of a mirror in normal stance (**A–D**), on tip-toes (**B**), on the heels (**C**)

17. The patient looks for three targets sited, respectively, in front of him, on his left and on his right. He fixates the front target, then he rapidly moves his head fixating the right-hand target. He then turns his head leftward maintaining the fixation of the right-hand target. The patient fixates the front target and then moves his head rapidly leftward and fixates the left-hand target. Then he turns his head rightward maintaining the fixation of the left-hand target.

18. The patient fixates himself in a mirror and correctly aligns his posture (Fig. 4.114A). He maintains equilibrium for 1 min and then he closes his eyes visualizing his correct position remaining in this position for at least 1 min. He then lifts himself up on his tiptoes maintaining equilibrium first with the eyes open fixating a mirror and then with the eyes closed (Fig. 4.114B). Then he lifts himself up on his heels maintaining equilibrium first with the eyes open fixating a mirror and then with the eyes closed (Fig. 4.114C). Finally, he returns to the resting position standing quietly in front of the mirror (Fig. 4.114C).

19. The patient moves up and down a step, fixating a target according to the following sequence:
Right foot up left foot up right foot down
Left foot down left foot up right foot up
Left foot down right foot down

He then repeats the exercise with the eyes closed.

20. Using the Rettiks

   a) The patient fixates himself in a mirror and correctly aligns his posture. He maintains equilibrium for 1 min and then he closes his eyes visualizing his correct position and remains in this position for at least 1 min (Fig. 4.115A). Then he oscillates rhythmically laterally (Fig. 4.115B). In succession he resists the attempts of the therapist to push him (Fig. 4.115C) and he maintains equilibrium crossing the legs (Fig. 4.115D).

   b) The patient fixates himself in a mirror, then oscillates to and fro and right and left around his ankles keeping his pelvis still (ankle strategy) (Fig. 4.116A).

   c) The patient fixates himself in a mirror; keeping the feet still he bends his trunk to and fro and right and left (hip strategy) (Fig. 4.116B).

   d) The patient grasps a stick (Fig. 4.117A) and then he lifts it over his head fixating it (Fig. 4.117B).

   e) The patient holds a small object and lifts it over his head fixating it. Then he inhales. Exhaling, he bends himself forward placing the object on the floor. He waits 10 s and then, inhaling, he lifts the object again over his head (Fig. 4.118).

   f) The parts of the mattress are placed in order to form a pathway. The patient walks to and fro with eyes open, fixating a target (Fig. 4.119).

21. Using the Skitter

   a) The patient steps on footpads with the feet centrally positioned. Then he concentrates on a proper posture using a mirror to see his reflection and transfers his weight from one foot to the other with a smooth flowing motion. During this smooth and rhythmic weight transfer the therapist induces body movements according to ankle or hip strategies (Fig. 4.120).

   b) The patient stands in a comfortable and stable position on the footpads. With his thumbs and limbs extended he tries to touch some visual targets placed in different positions on a facing mirror.

22. Using the Daedalus: The patient sits comfortably and maneuvers the ball through the labyrinth. The position of the patient on the chair can be modified in order to improve the trunk antigravitational muscles (trunk slightly bent forward) or leg muscles (patient's back resting against the chair back) (Fig. 4.121).

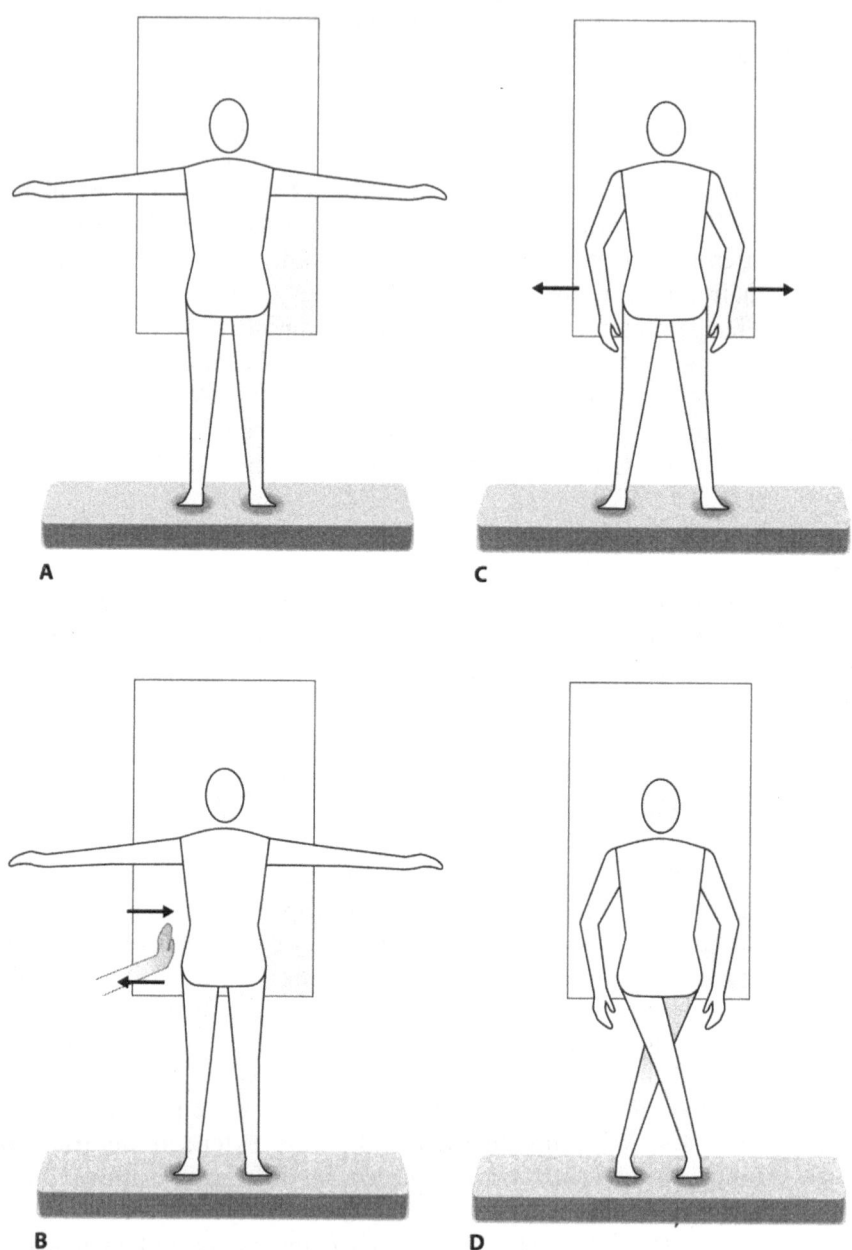

Fig. 4.115A–D. Standing on a mattress the patient controls his posture

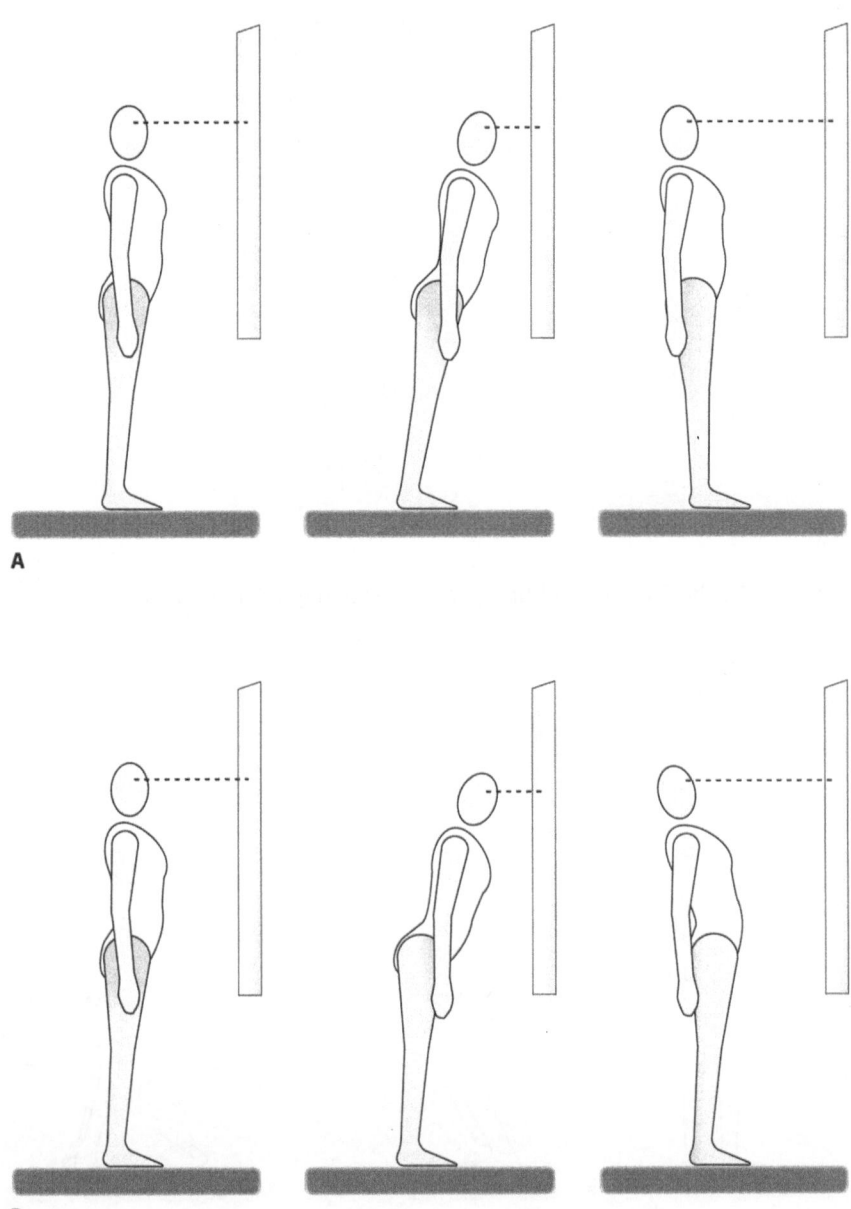

Fig. 4.116. A Ankle oscillations and **B** hip oscillations, standing on a mattress

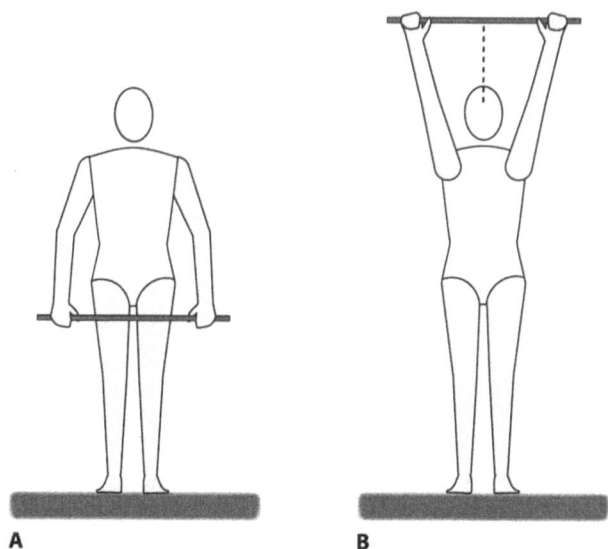

Fig. 4.117A, B. Grasping and lifting a stick, standing on a mattress

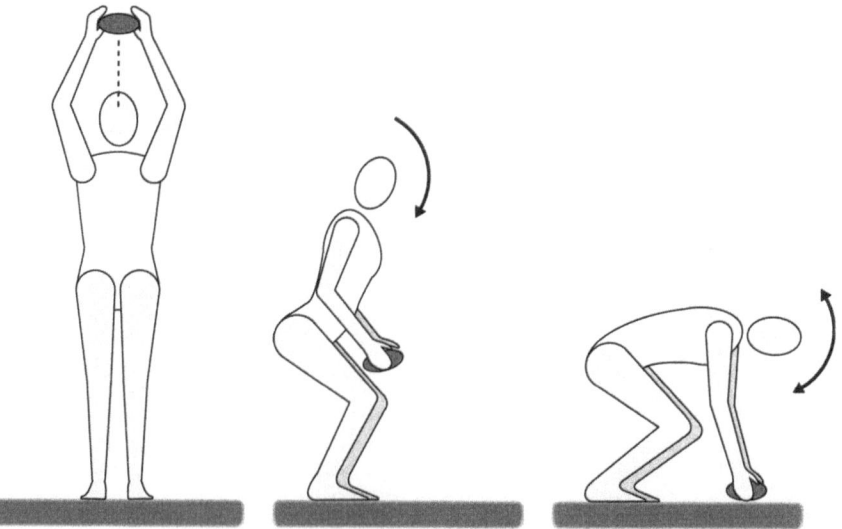

Fig. 4.118. Fixating an object and then placing it on the floor, standing on a mattress

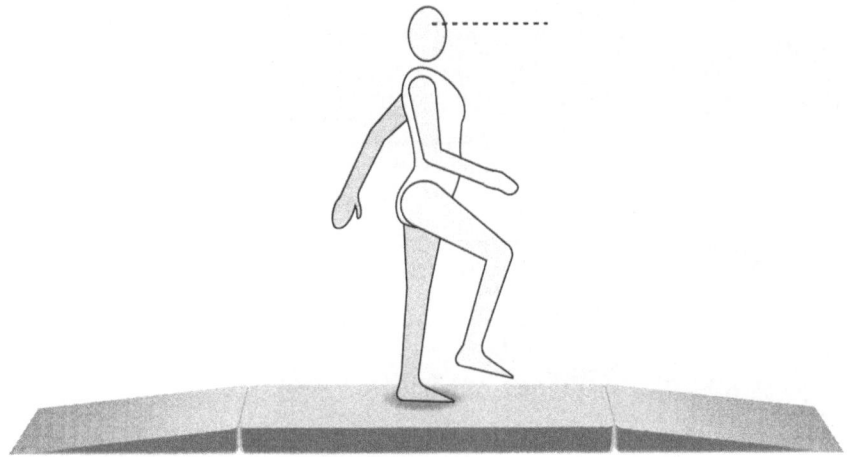

Fig. 4.119. Walking on the Rettiks mattress

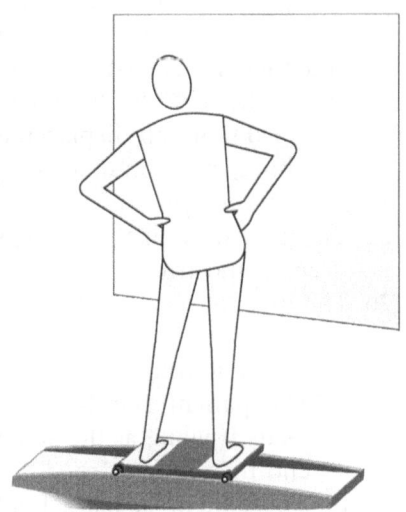

Fig. 4.120. Smooth weight changes on the Skitter fixating a mirror

Synergetics Phase

In this phase the exercises must be performed during VES. If vestibular hypofunction has been documented, electrodes need to be placed according to the side of hypofunction. In the other cases electrodes need to be placed symmetrically on both sides of the neck. If possible, exercises should be performed with the patient wearing prisms (3°) with both bases facing outwards in order to stimulate vergence.

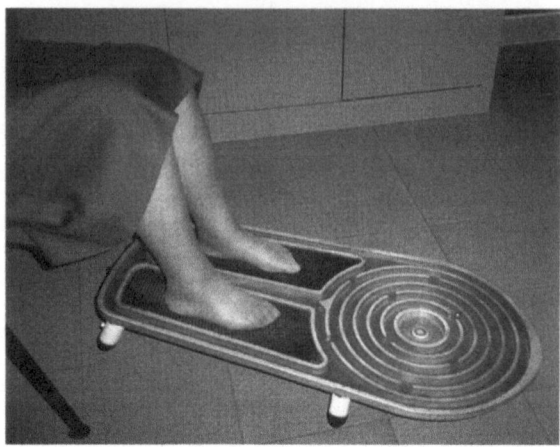

Fig. 4.121. Using the Daedalus in the sitting position

23. The patient extends his right arm and lifts his thumb. He moves slowly his arm to and fro slowly first in a horizontal direction and then in a vertical direction. He follows his thumb with the eyes only, first slowly and then increasing progressively the velocity of the thumb displacement.
24. As above, but simultaneously moving also the head while trying to keep the eyes still.
25. The patient walks five steps forward and backward moving his head to and fro.
26. The patient walks five steps forward and backward reading a book.
27. Using the Rettiks
    a) The patient stands, then opens a book in front of him. He reads it while at the same time moving the book right and left and then to and fro.
    b) The patient opens a book in front of him and then moves it away from him extending his arms. He reads it, then brings it closer to him, slowly, trying to read it. Then he moves it away again and repeats the exercise several times to and fro.
    c) The patient performs steps moving the head to and fro.
    d) The patient performs steps reading a book.
28. Using the Daedalus.
    a) The patient stands comfortably on the platform. He tries maintaining equilibrium during smooth pursuit of a small target (e.g., a small ball or the finger of the therapist) moving in front of him (Fig. 4.122).

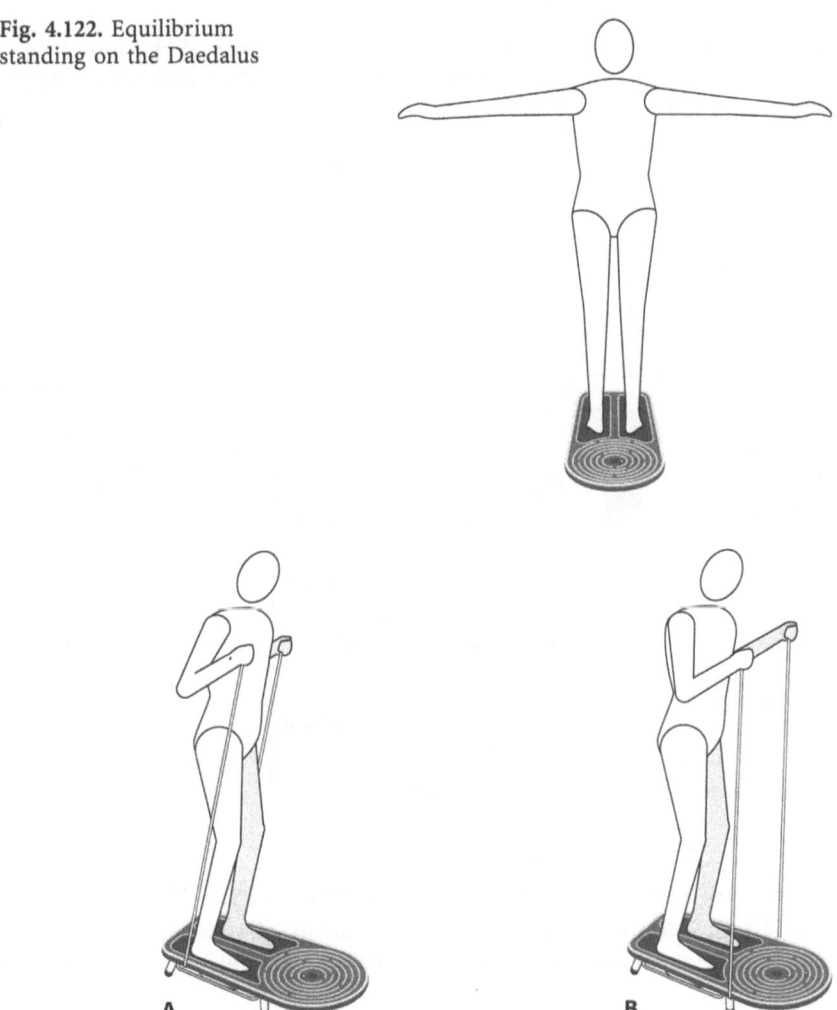

Fig. 4.122. Equilibrium standing on the Daedalus

A   B

Fig. 4.123A, B. Patient maneuvers a ball through the labyrinth grasping the sticks

b) The patient stands on the platform, grasping the sticks both placed posteriorly, and he maneuvers the ball through the labyrinth (Fig. 4.123A): then he maneuvers the ball through the labyrinth grasping the sticks placed anteriorly (Fig. 4.123B).

28. By visual feedback: the position of the target is generally that which reproduces the perimeter of the limits of stability. To improve hip strategy the target is placed in a small circle with a fast pacing (5 s or less) (Fig. 4.124), while to improve ankle strategy it

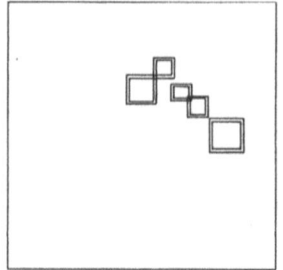

Fig. 4.124. Close arrangement of different-sized targets (Balance Master, reproduced by courtesy of NeuroCom International, Inc., Clackamas, Oregon, USA)

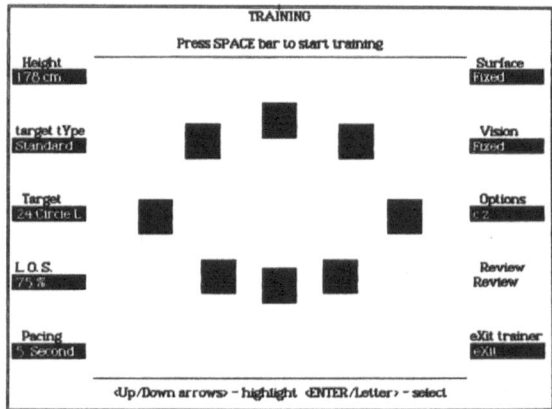

Fig. 4.125. Wide arrangement of targets along the perimeter of stability (Balance Master, reproduced by courtesy of NeuroCom International, Inc., Clackamas, Oregon, USA)

has to be placed in a larger circle (Fig. 4.125) with a slow pacing (10 s). According to previous evaluation of the patient, the target may placed especially in the anterior, posterior or lateral positions.

Home Protocol

The exercises are subdivided according to the different phases of equilibrium, from supine to standing to moving. In each phase, there is a progression from mechanics to synergetics exercises. The exercises must be as simple as possible to ensure both continuous daily repetition and maintenance of the results obtained with the therapist in the gymnasium.

Home exercises can never be substituted for the therapeutic programs described in the previous section, performed with the therapist. Home exercises are used to complete the therapy. All the protocols have to be performed for 2 weeks, possibly twice a day. After 2 weeks the program can be reduced to the following exercises: 4, 6, 9, 13, 14, 15, 19, 20, 25, 30.

A. Supine

1. Hold your right knee against the chest, then extend your leg and hold your left knee against the chest. When you hold the knee against the chest softly traction the flexed leg with the hands.
2. Extend your left arm over your head and simultaneously hold the right flexed leg to the chest, helping with your hand. Maintain this position for 10 s and then repeat using the opposite arm and leg.
3. Lift your left leg with the extended knee and then repeat with your right leg.
4. Grasp a stick. Take your extended arms over your head and then return to the starting position.
5. Fixate a target on the ceiling and slowly move your head rightward and leftward.
6. Look for two equidistant targets on the ceiling and then fixate them alternatively first moving only the eyes and then moving only the head.
7. Turn your head rightward and fixate a target on the lateral wall. Then straighten your head straight maintaining the visual fixation. Count up to 10 and then turn your head.
8. Turn your head leftward and fix a target on the lateral wall. Then straighten your head straight maintaining the visual fixation. Count up to 10 and then turn your head.
9. From the supine position move to the sitting position fixating a point straight in front of you.
10. In the prone position lift your left arm and right leg maintaining your forehead over the bed. Then repeat with the right arm and the left leg.
11. Repeat as above but at the same time also lifting the head.

B. Sitting

12. Extend your arms and lift your thumbs. Move your arms along a horizontal plane at about 50 cm from your eyes and then fixate your thumbs alternately. Begin slowly and then increase progressively the velocity of alternate fixation.
13. Extend your arms and lift your thumbs. Move your arms along a vertical plane at about 50 cm from your eyes and then fixate your thumbs alternately. Begin slowly and then increase progressively the velocity of alternate fixation.

14. Extend your right arm and lift your thumb. Move your arm slowly to and fro first in a horizontal direction and then in a vertical direction. Follow your thumb with the eyes only, first slowly and then increasing progressively the velocity of thumb displacement.

15. As above but simultaneously moving also the head while trying to keep the eyes still.

16. Move your head first slowly and then more rapidly in all directions fixating a target straight in front of you.

17. Look for three targets sited, respectively, in front of you, on your left and on your right. Fixate the front target, then move your head rapidly fixating the right-hand target. Now rotate your head leftward maintaining the fixation of the right-hand target. Fixate the frontal target. Now rapidly move your head leftward and fixate the left-hand target. Then rotate your head rightward maintaining the fixation of the left-hand target.

18. Open a book in front of you. Move it away from you extending your arms. Read it. Then move it closer to you, slowly, trying to read it. Then move it away. Repeat several times to and fro.

C. Standing

19. With your hands on a table lift yourself on your tiptoes and maintain this position for 30 s.

20. With your hands on a table lift yourself on your heels and maintain this position for 30 s.

21. Fixate yourself in a mirror. Align your position correctly. Maintain equilibrium for 1 min and then close your eyes visualizing your correct position and remain in this position for at least 1 min.

22. Fixate yourself in a mirror. Then oscillate to and fro and right and left, around your ankles keeping your pelvis still.

23. Fixate yourself in a mirror; keeping your feet still, bend your trunk to and fro and right and left.

24. Hold a small object and then lift it over your head and fixate it. With your arms extended move it in circles of increasing width maintaining the fixation of the object.

25. Open a book in front of you. Move it away from you extending your arms. Read it. Then move it near to you, slowly, trying to read it. Then move it away. Repeat several times to and fro.

D. Moving

26. Stepping on the floor with the eyes open fixating a target straight in front of you.

27. Support yourself on a chair and then step on the tiptoes.

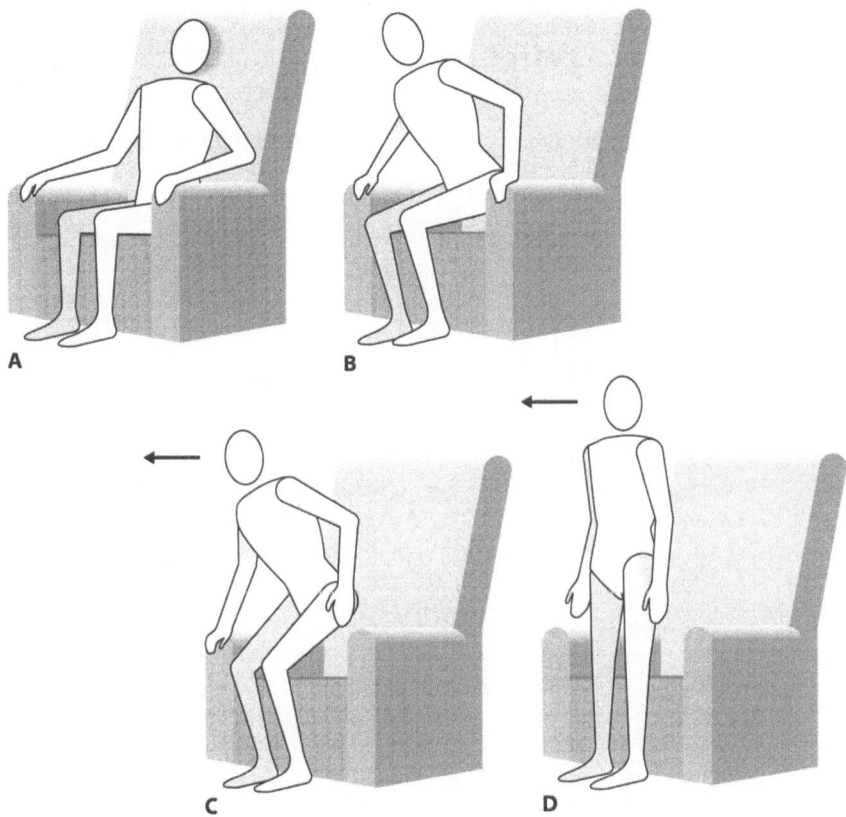

Fig. 4.126A–D. How to get up from a chair

28. Support yourself on a chair and then step on the heels.
29. Walk for five steps along a corridor forward and backward fixating a target.
30. Walk for five steps along a corridor forward and backward moving your head to and fro.
31. Walk for five steps along a corridor forward and backward reading a book.

Some Suggestions To Ameliorate Lifestyle

A. How to get up from a chair
  1. Place your hands on the chair arms (Fig. 4.126A).
  2. Bend your trunk forward and lift yourself pushing on the chair arms (Fig. 4.126B).

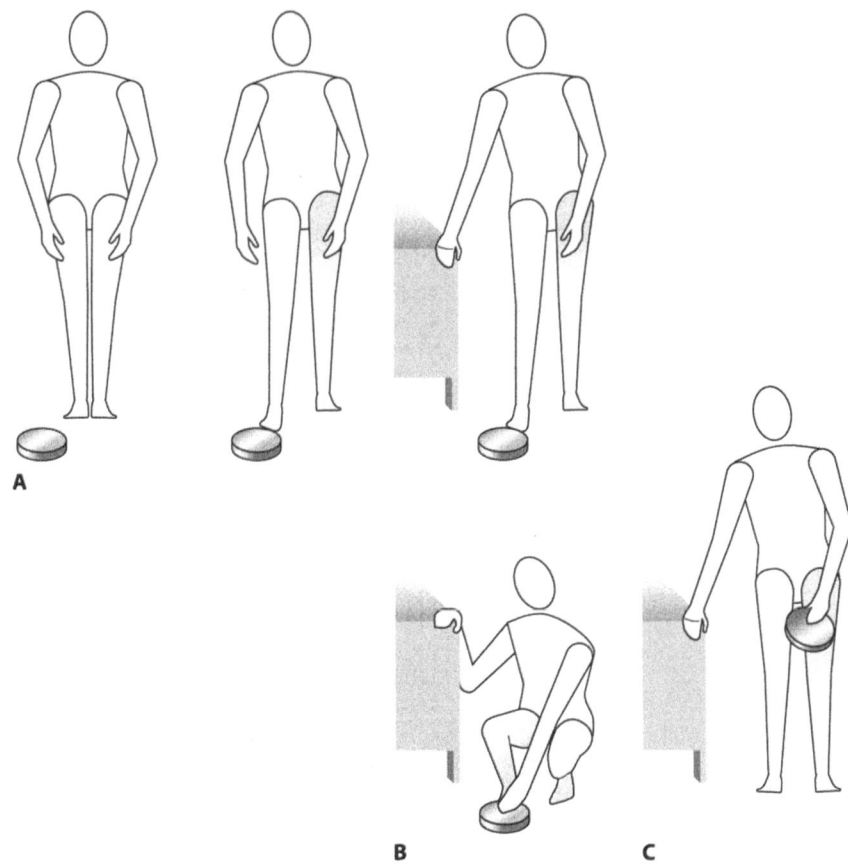

Fig. 4.127A–C. How to pick up an object

3. Now get up fixating in front of you (Fig. 4.126C).
4. Wait a few seconds before walking and continue to fixate in front of you (Fig. 4.126D).

B. How to pick up an object from the floor
1. Push the object near a table or a similar object (Fig. 4.127A).
2. Using the table for support, bend yourself at the knees and pick up the object (Fig. 4.127B).
3. Lift yourself using the table for support (Fig. 4.127C).

C How to get out of bed
1. Turn yourself onto one side (Fig. 4.128B).
2. Move your legs over the side of the bed (Fig. 4.128C).
3. Lift your trunk slowly (Fig. 4.128D).

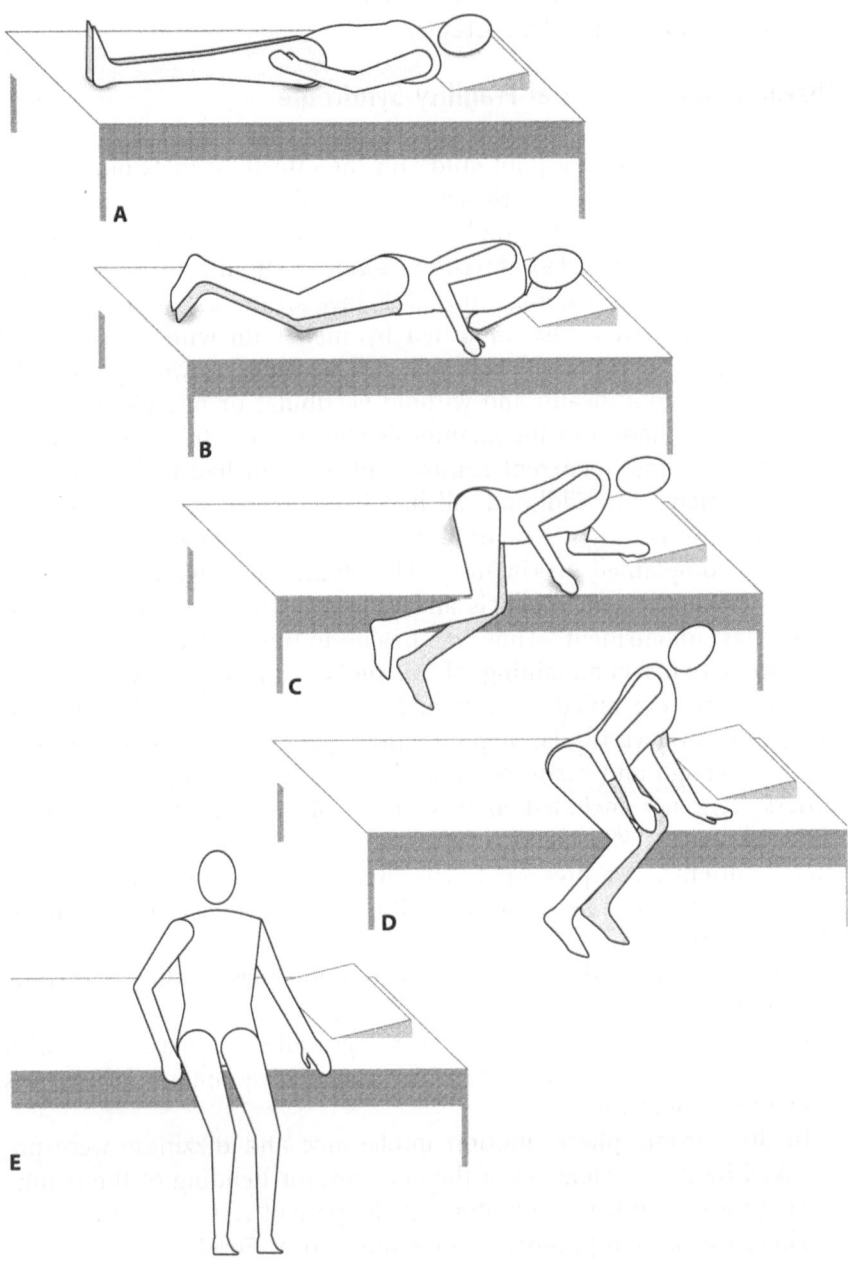

Fig. 4.128A–E. How to get out of bed

4. Sit fixating in front of you, remaining still for a few seconds before standing up (Fig. 4.128D).

Dizziness and Structural Fragility Syndrome

During the course of a pilot study on the effects of melatonin on human equilibrium, we investigated 13 normal volunteers. Both electro-oculography and posturography were performed. The administration of a single dose of melatonin 10 mg induced significant modifications of posturographic findings in all subjects. In six subjects oculographic results were also modified by melatonin with a decrease in saccadic and pursuit performances. All the subjects were young (23–28 years), in good health and without vestibular or neurological problems. A reevaluation of the anamnesis showed that five out of six presented with some recurrent features: all of them had had scoliosis or spine problems in childhood, all had been treated for occlusal disorders, all showed slight ocular problems such as heterophoria and all of them complained of kinetosis. This evidence suggests that heterophoria, malocclusion, scoliosis and kinetosis are disorders facilitating vestibular impairment. Thus we began to investigate these aspects also in patients complaining of vertigo or dizziness. Over the past year we have examined a series of 2357 dizzy patients. Meniere's disease, unilateral vestibular hypofunction, positional vertigo, any other kind of vertigo and easily recognizable vestibular or neurological disorders were not included in this group of subjects. Over a third of these patients (37%) could be classified as "functional" or psychosomatic patients. All presented with heterophoria, scoliosis, kinetosis and occlusal problems combined with neuro-otological recurrent and characteristic features:

- They presented with a vague sense of dizziness rather than frank vertigo.
- In the acute phase symptoms were typically provoked by head or body movements without typical signs and symptoms of paroxysmal positional vertigo.
- In the chronic phase, motion intolerance and dizziness were provoked by flexo-extension of the head and/or bending of the trunk.
- There were remitting symptoms if the patient remained still.
- There was a high proportion of women (over 70%).
- A double peak in the age distribution was revealed: 25–28 years and the menopausal period.

Also instrumental findings were recurrent:
- Normal saccades.
- Low smooth pursuit gain (0.6–0.65).
- Low optokinetic nystagmus gain.
- Slight labyrinth hyporeflexia with qualitative alterations of nystagmus beats.
- Better posturographic performance with eyes closed than with eyes open (so-called postural blindness).
- Mixed craniocorpographic pattern with slight incoordination of the head-trunk relationship.

In conclusion, we presume that kinetosis, heterophoria, scoliosis and malocclusion represent structural elements that disturb normal vestibular function and can facilitate dizziness. The specific treatment must be aimed at the most relevant problem of the specific patient: treatment of occlusal problems, orthotic reeducation, antihistamines for kinetosis or scoliosis reeducation. In all cases an associated vestibular rehabilitation program is useful.

Rehabilitation has to be aimed at:
1. Enforcement of antigravitational muscles.
2. Relaxation of cervicodorsal muscles.
3. Activation of visual fixation, because, usually, these patients have problems in utilization of mechanisms of fixation.
4. Recalibration of sensorial preference.

Exercises in the Gymnasium

Mechanics Phase
1. The patient lifts his left leg, extending the knee, he maintains this position for 10 s and then he extends the right knee (Fig. 4.129).

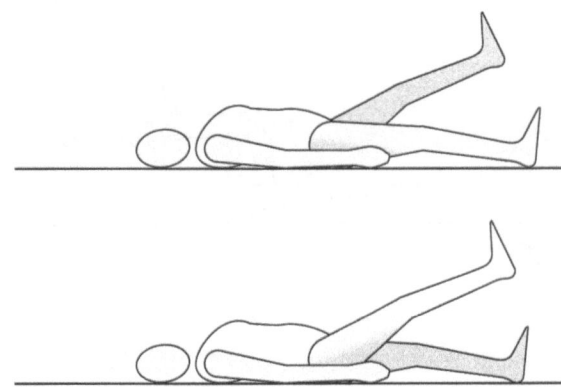

Fig. 4.129. Extension of the knees

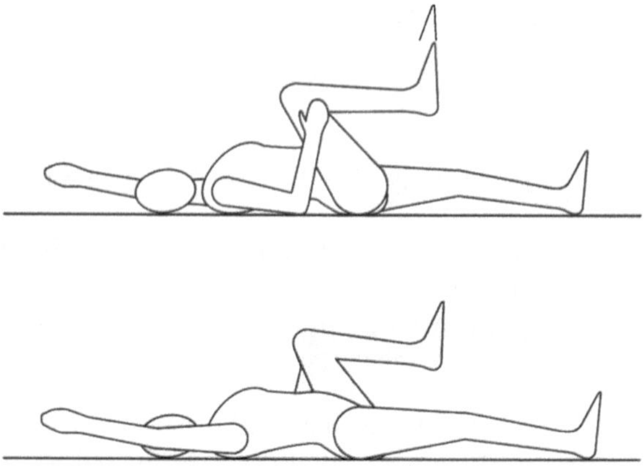

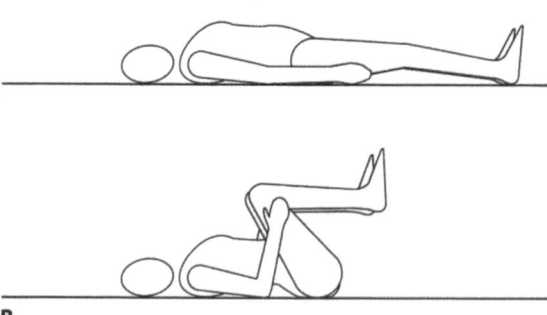

Fig. 4.130. Flexion of the knee with simultaneous extension of the opposite arm

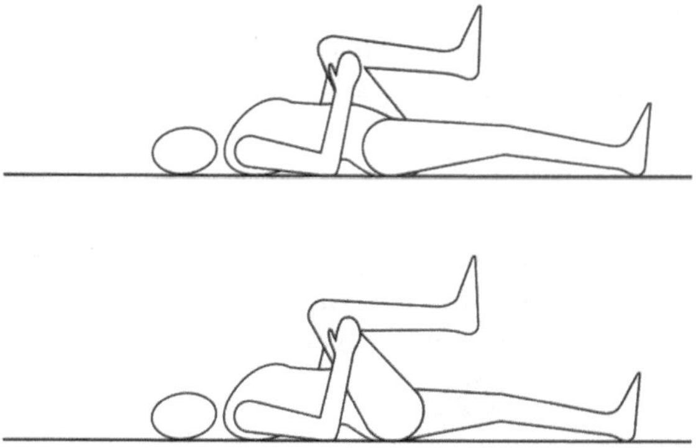

Fig. 4.131A, B. Exercises with the knees for the pelvis

A

B
B

Fig. 4.132. Arm-leg synchronization

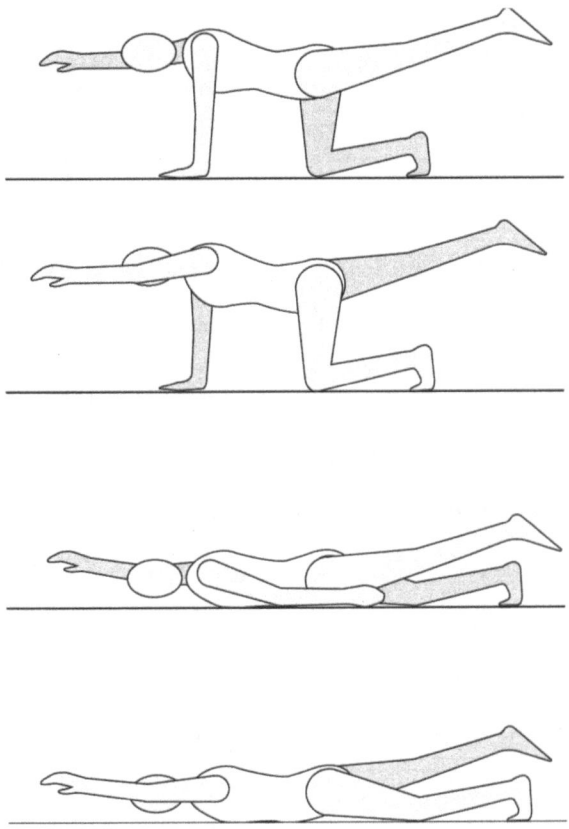

2. The patient extends his left arm over his head and simultaneously
   moves the right flexed leg to the chest, helping with his hand. He
   maintains this position for 10 s and then repeats with the opposite
   arm and leg (Fig. 4.130).
3. The patient holds his left leg against the chest with the flexed
   knee, maintaining this position for 10 s and then he repeats the
   exercise with the right leg. He then holds both knees against the
   chest (Fig. 4.131).
4. In the quadrupedal position he extends the right arm and the left
   leg and then he repeats with the opposite arm and leg. He then repeats this exercise in the prone position (Fig. 4.132).
5. The patient, with his hands on a chair, lifts himself onto his tiptoes, maintaining this position for 30 s (Fig. 4.133A).
6. The patient, with his hands on a chair, lifts himself on his heels,
   maintaining this position for 30 s (Fig. 4.133B).

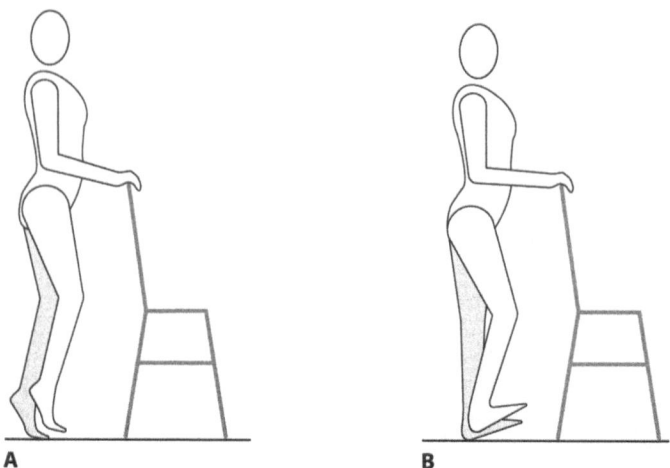

Fig. 4.133A, B. Equilibrium on tiptoes and heels

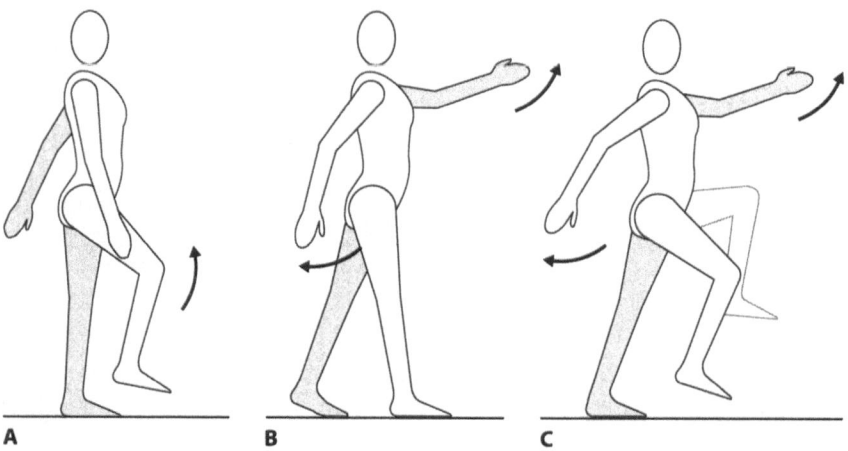

Fig. 4.134. A Stepping; **B** oscillations of the arms; **C** stepping with simultaneous oscillations of the arms

7. The patient performs a stepping movement (Fig. 4.134A) with the arms still.
8. The patient oscillates his arms rhythmically as during gait (Fig. 4.134B).
9. He then repeats the stepping movement oscillating the arms at the same time (Fig. 4.134C).
10. Using the Skitter

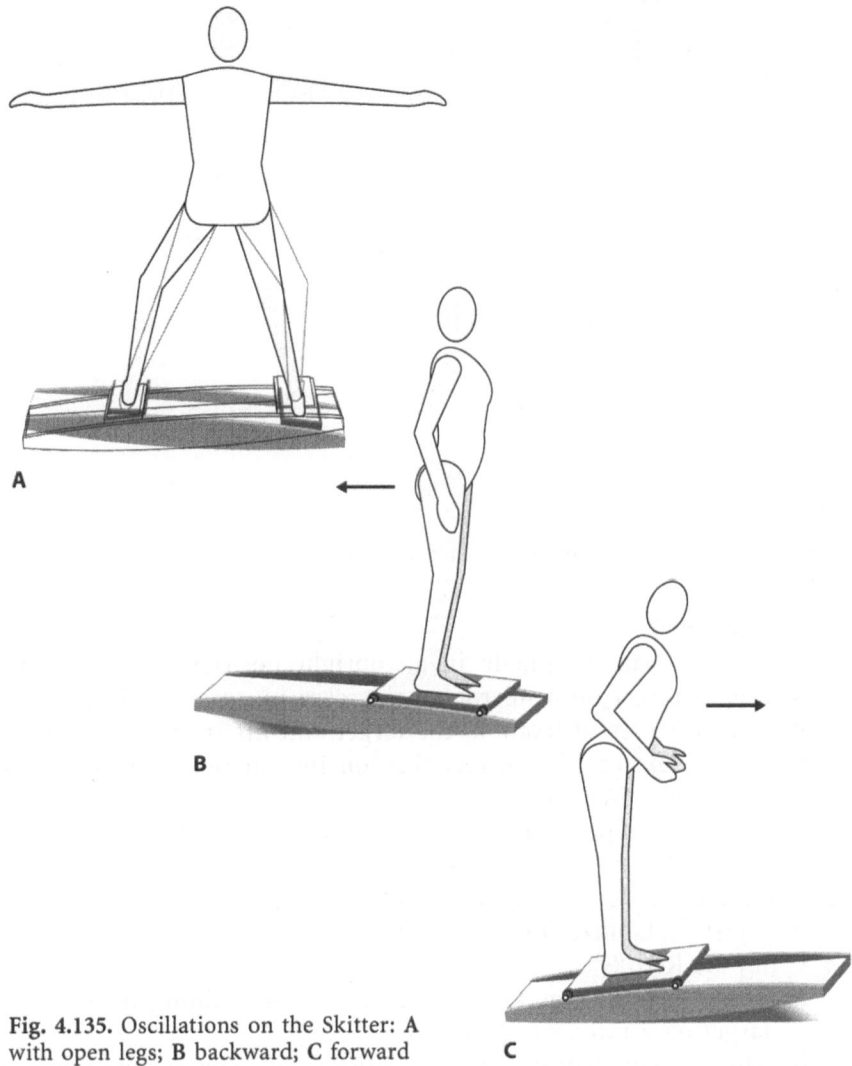

Fig. 4.135. Oscillations on the Skitter: A with open legs; **B** backward; **C** forward

a) The patient swings around rhythmically on the device maintaining equilibrium with the arms (Fig. 4.135A).
b) The patient oscillates himself in a backward direction standing on one of the ends of the device (Fig. 4.135B).
c) The patient oscillates himself in a forward direction standing on the other end of the device (Fig. 4.135C).

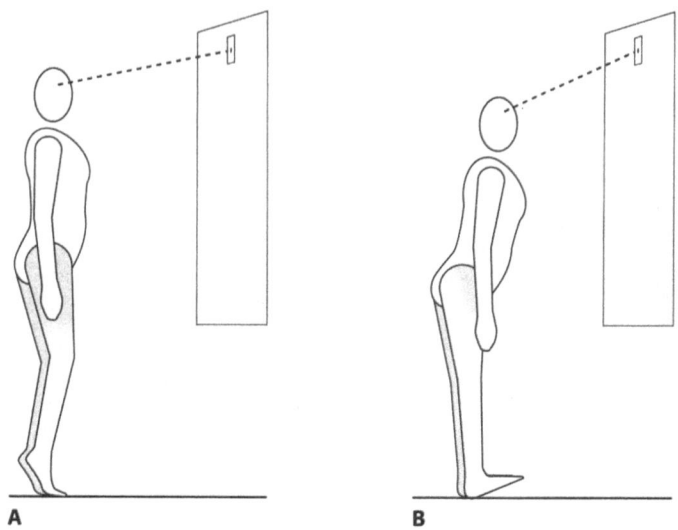

Fig. 4.136. Exercises on tiptoes (**A**) and heels (**B**) fixating a target on a mirror

Cybernetics Phase

1. The patient stands quietly in an upright position on tiptoes and fixating a target on a mirror. In this case he receives visual inputs from two planes of fixation: the target and his image. He needs to be able to extract the correct fixation information from visual inputs (Fig. 4.136A).
2. The patient repeats the same exercise standing on the heels (Fig. 4.136B).
3. The patient rides a cylinder fixating a target on a mirror and the therapist destabilizes him (Fig. 4.137).
4. Using the Rettiks
   a) The patient swings around his ankles maintaining fixation of a target on a mirror (Fig. 4.138A).
   b) The patient repeats the oscillations but now using the hips (Fig. 4.138B).
   c) The patient holds a small object over his head. Fixating it, he moves the object in small circles. Then, maintaining circular movements of the object and its fixation, he bends himself placing the object on the floor (Fig. 4.139).
   d) The patient maintains equilibrium in different conditions, fixating a target on a mirror (Fig. 4.140): quietly standing (A), crossing his legs (B), resisting the therapist's destabilization (C) and standing on one leg (D).

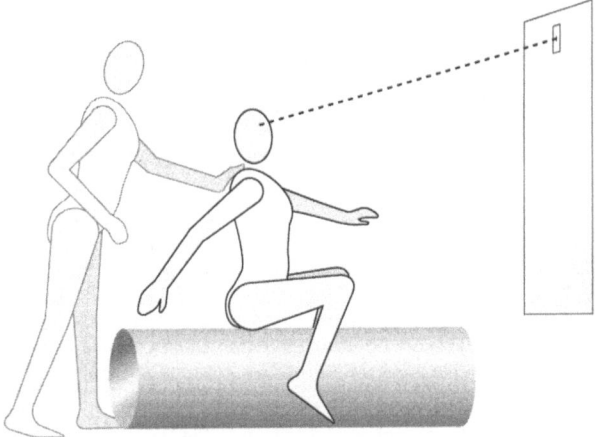

Fig. 4.137. Equilibrium riding a cylinder fixating a target on a mirror

  e) The patient synchronizes arms and legs (Fig. 4.141): in the quadrupedal position (A) and standing on the mattress during stepping (B): it is better if two parts of the mattress have been overlapped.
  f) The three parts of the mattress constitute a route. The patient runs along it fixating a target on a mirror (Fig. 4.142).
5. Using the Daedalus: the patient stands quietly on the platform and rhythmically oscillates his arms, maintaining equilibrium. It is better if he fixates a target on a mirror (Fig. 4.143).
6. Using the Skitter: the patient swing himself on the device as in slalom, fixating a target on a mirror (Fig. 4.144).

Synergetics Phase
1. Using the Rettiks: the patient stands quietly on the mattress. In front of him there is a mirror with several targets placed in different positions. Following the therapist's orders he has to point to one target as fast as possible (Fig. 4.145).
2. Using the Daedalus: quietly standing on the platform the patient maneuvers the ball through the labyrinth, wearing 3° outward-based prisms (Fig. 4.146).
3. By Stabilometry: the patient moves his CoG towards an anterior target placed as in Figs. 4.147 and 4.148, wearing 3° outward-based prisms.

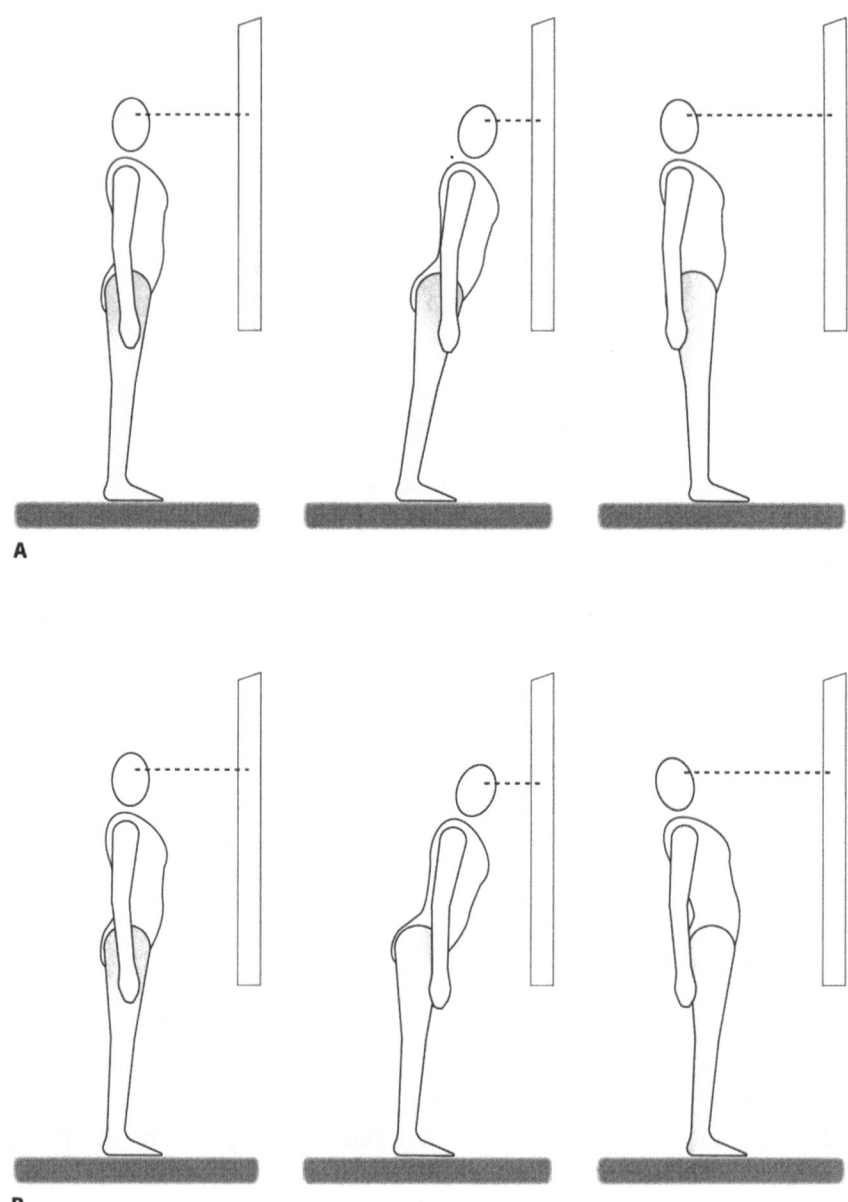

Fig. 4.138. Ankle (A) and hip (B) oscillations standing on a mattress

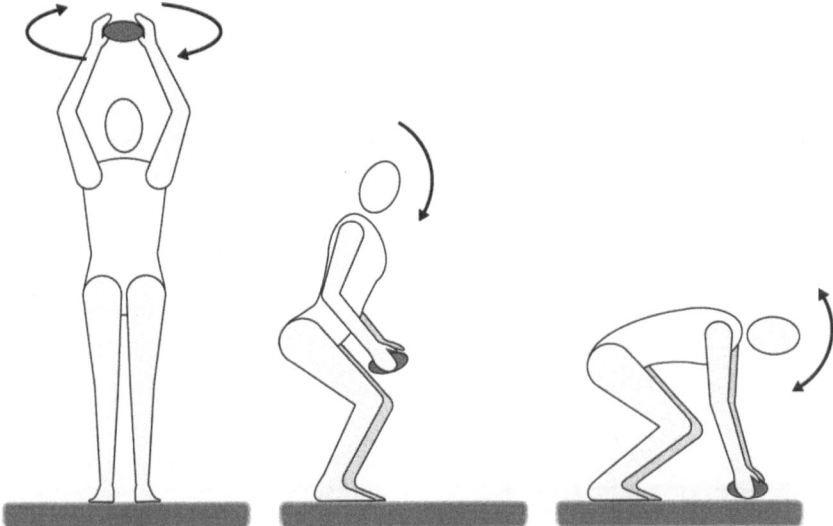

Fig. 4.139. Lifting over the head an object and turning it, during fixation. The patient then places it on the floor

Home Protocol

The exercises are subdivided according to different phases of equilibrium, passing from supine to standing to moving. In each phase, there is a progression from mechanics to synergetics exercises. Home exercises can never substitute for the therapeutic programs shown in the previous section, performed with the therapist. Home exercises complete the therapeutic program and maintain the results obtained.

A. Supine
1. Extend your left arm over your head and at the same time hold the right flexed leg to the chest, helping with your hand. Maintain this position for 10 s and then repeat inverting the arm and leg.
2. Lift your left leg with the extended knee.
3. Lift your right leg with the extended knee.
4. Repeat with the tip of the foot outward.
5. Repeat with the tip of the foot inward.
6. Fixate a target on the ceiling and slowly move your head rightward and leftward.
7. Look for two equidistant targets on the ceiling and then fixate them alternately first moving only the eyes and then moving only the head.

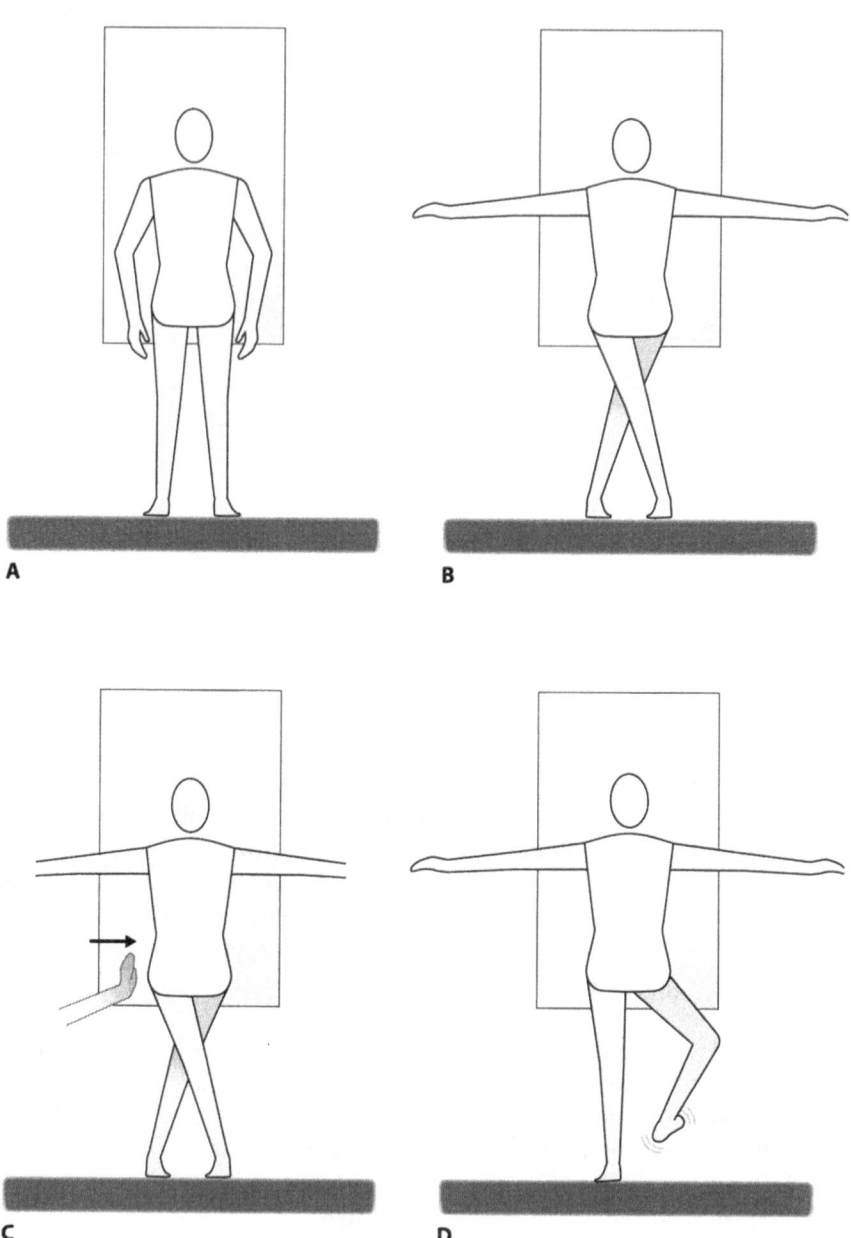

Fig. 4.140A–D. Equilibrium exercises on the mattress

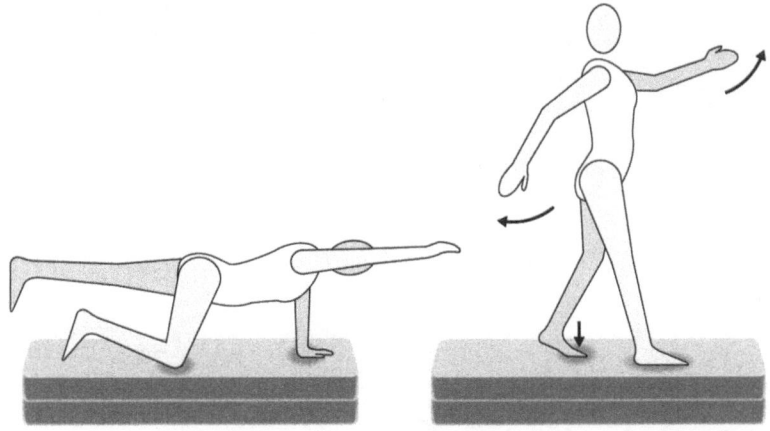

Fig. 4.141. Arm-leg synchronization on the mattress

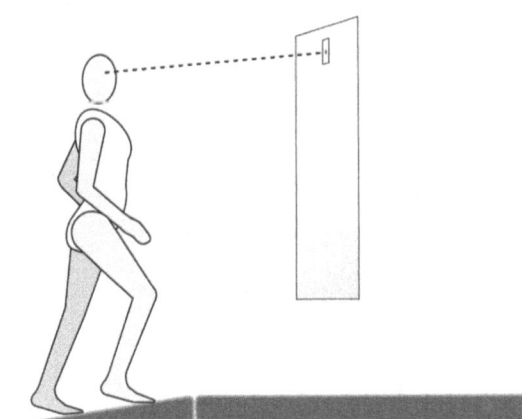

Fig. 4.142. Walking on
the mattress fixating a
target on the mirror

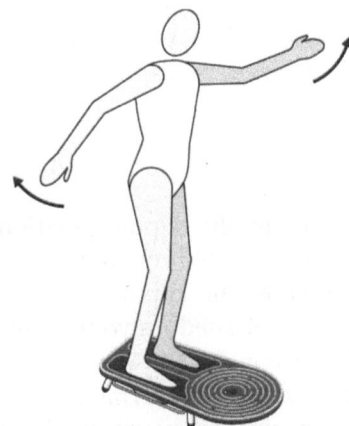

Fig. 4.143. Rhythmic oscillation on the
Daedalus

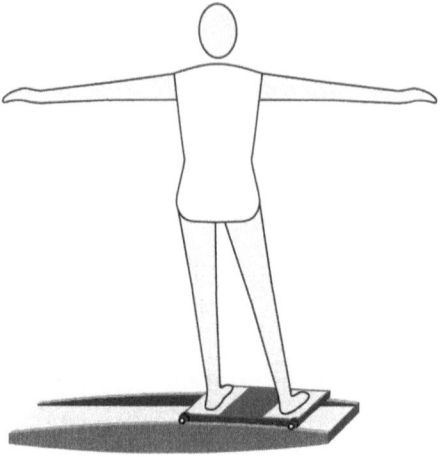

Fig. 4.144. Slalom-like oscillation on the Skitter

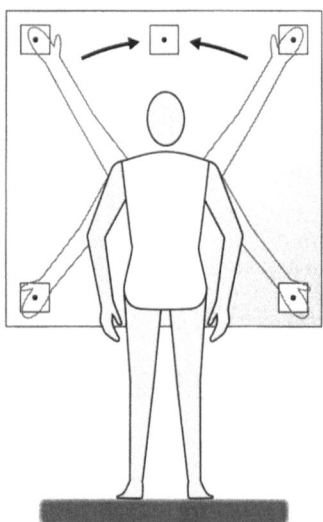

Fig. 4.145. Pointing to different targets on a mirror, standing on the mattress

8. From the supine position move to the sitting position fixating a target sited on your left.
9. From the supine position move to the sitting position fixating a target sited on your right.

B. Sitting

10. Extend your arms and lift your thumbs. Move your arms along a horizontal plane at about 50 cm from your eyes and then fixate

Fig. 4.146. Maneuvering a ball through the labyrinth

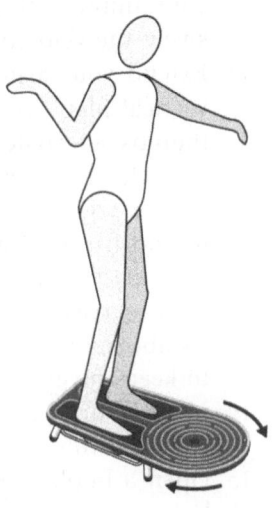

Fig. 4.147. Stabilometric visual feedback exercise to improve the back antigravitational muscles, which is performed wearing 3° outward-based prisms (Balance Master, reproduced by courtesy of Neuro-Com International, Inc, Clackamas, Oregon, USA)

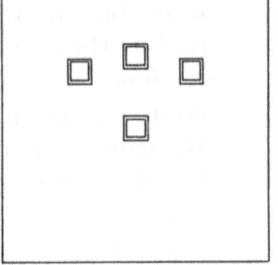

Fig. 4.148. Stabilometric visual feedback exercise to improve anteroposterior sway, which is performed wearing 3° outward-based prisms (Balance Master, reproduced by courtesy of NeuroCom International, Inc, Clackamas, Oregon, USA)

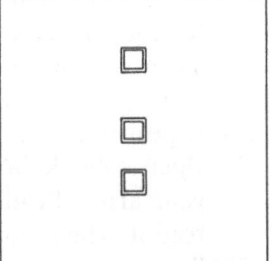

your thumbs alternately. Begin slowly and then increase progressively the velocity of alternate fixation.

11. Extend your arms and lift your thumbs. Move your arms along a vertical plane at about 50 cm from your eyes and then fixate your thumbs alternately. Begin slowly and then increase progressively the velocity of alternate fixation.

12. Extend your right arm and lift your thumb. Move your arm slowly to and fro first in a horizontal direction and then in a vertical direction. Follow your thumb with the eyes only, first slowly and then increasing progressively the velocity of thumb displacement.

13. As above but at the same time also moving the head while trying to keep the eyes still.

14. Move your head first slowly and then more rapidly in all directions fixating a target straight in front of you placed on a mirror.

15. Open a book in front of you. Read it moving, simultaneously, the book right and left and then to and fro.

16. Open a book in front of you. Move it away from you extending your arms. Read it. Then move it closer to you, slowly, trying to read it. Then move it away. Repeat several times to and fro.

C. Standing

17. Fixate a target placed on a mirror. Align your position correctly. Maintain equilibrium for 1 min and then close your eyes visualizing your correct position and remain in this position for at least 1 min.

18. Repeat the same exercise standing on a soft mattress.

19. Fixate a target placed on a mirror. Then oscillate to and fro and right and left, around your ankles keeping your pelvis still.

20. Fixate a target placed on a mirror; keeping your feet still, bend your trunk to and fro and right and left.

21. Repeat exercises 19 and 20 standing on a soft mattress.

22. Open a book in front of you. Read it while moving it to and fro and right and left.

23. Repeat this exercise on a soft mattress.

24. Open a book in front of you. Move it away from you extending your arms. Read it. Then move it closer to you, slowly, trying to read it. Then move it away. Repeat several times.

25. Repeat on a soft mattress.

D. Moving

26. Stepping, fixate a target placed on a mirror in front of you.

27. Stepping, read a book.

28. Stepping on a soft mattress, read a book.

29. Walk for five steps along a corridor forward and backward while fixating a target.
30. Walk for five steps along a corridor forward and backward moving your head to and fro, maintaining your fixation of a target.
31. Walk for five steps along a corridor forward and backward while reading a book.

After the 1st week of home treatment, the protocol is reduced to the synergetics exercises to be performed at least once a day: 12, 15, 16, 18, 19, 20, 21, 25, 28, 30.

Bibliography

Alpini D (1994) The Italian Vestibular Rehabilitation Protocols. Neurol Newslett 1:54–66

Alpini D, Cesarani A, Barozzi S (1992) Nonpharmacological treatment of acute vertigo. In: Claussen CF, Kirtane MV, Schneider D (eds) Diagnostic procedures and imaging techniques used in neurotology. Proceedings of the XVI NES Congress, Dr. Werner Rudat & Co. Nachf. Edn. M+P, Hamburg, pp 337–340

Alpini D, Pugnetti L, Cesarani A, Mendozzi L, Barbieri E (1996) Evaluation of vestibular strategies in human exploration of the environment by means of immersive virtual reality. In: Claussen CF, Constantinescu L, Kirtane MV, Schneider D (eds) Proceedings of the NES, vol XXIV, Elsevier Science BV, Amsterdam, pp 315–323

Asai M, Watanabe Y, Shimizu K (1997) Effects of vestibular rehabilitation on postural control. Acta Otolaryngol (Suppl 528):116–120

Ashby WR (1956) An introduction to cybernetics. Chapman & Hall, London

Balk JH, Picetti R, Salardi A, Thirlet G, Dierich A, Depaulis A, Le Meur M, Borrelli E (1995) Parkinsonian-like locomotor impairment in mice lacking dopamine D2 receptors. Nature 377:424–428

Barany R (1906) Untersuchungen über den vom Vestibularapparat des Ohres reflektorisch ausgelösten rhythmischen Nystagmus und seine Begleiterscheinung. Mschr Ohrenheilk 40:193–297

Barany R, Wittmaack K (1911) Funktionelle Prüfung des Vestibularapparates. Fischer-Verlag, Jena

Baron JB (1963) Correction prismatique dans les syndromes subjectifs post-commotionnels. Bulletin de la Societe Belge D'Ophtalmologie 133:246

Basar E(1980) EEG-brain dynamics. Elsevier Biomedical Press, Amsterdam

Bekkers JM (1993) Enhancement by histamine of NMDA-receptors synaptic transmission in the hippocampus. Science 261:104–106

Berg KO, Maki BE, Williams JI, Holliday PJ, Wood-Dauphinee SL (1992) Clinical and laboratory measures of postural balance in an elderly population. Arch Phys Med Rehabil 73:1073–1080

Bertalanffy Von L (1962) General system theory – a critical review. General System Yearbook 7:1–20

Berthoz A, Llinas R (1974) Afferent neck projection to the cat cerebellar cortex. Exp Brain Res 20:385–401

Biguer B, Donaldson IML, Hein A, Jannerod M (1988) Neck muscle vibration modifies the representation of visual motion and direction in man. Brain 111:1405–1424

Birsdoff A, Bronstein A, Gresty M, Wolsley C (1996) Subjective postural vertical inferred from vestibular-optokinetic vs proprioceptive cues. Brain Res Bull 40(5/6):413–415

Bles W, Roos JWP (1991) The tilting room and posturography. Acta Otorhinolaryngol Belg 45:387–391

Bohmer A, Mast F, Jarchow T (1996) Can a unilateral loss of otolithic function be clinically detected by assessment of the subjective visual vertical? Brain Res Bull 40(5/6):423–429

Boyle R, Pompeiano O (1981) Convergence and interaction of neck and macular vestibular inputs on vestibulospinal neurons. J Neurophysiol 45:852–866

Brink EE, Suzuki I, Timerick SJB, Wilson VJ (1985) Tonic neck reflex of the decerebrate cat: a role for propriospinal neurons. J Neurophysiol 54:978–987

Bronstein AM, Brandt T, Woollacott MH (eds) (1996) Clinical disorders of balance, posture and gait. Arnold Ed, London

Cass SP, Borellofrance D, Furman JM (1996) Functional outcome of vestibular rehabilitation in patients with abnormal sensory-organization testing. Am J Otology (N4):581–594

Cawthorne T (1944) The physiological basis of head exercises. J Chart Soc Physiother 106

Cesarani A (1994) The cervical electrostimulation. Neurootol Newslett 1(1):67–72

Cesarani A, Alpini D (1991) New trends in rehabilitation treatment of vertigo and dizziness. In: Akyildiz N, Portmann M (eds) Vertigo and its treatment. Proceedings of International Symposium for Prof. G. Portmann's Centenary, Ankara, 16–18 May 1990, Ankara, pp 90–104

Cesarani A, Alpini D (eds) (1994) Equilibrium disorders. Brainstem and cerebellar pathology. Springer-Verlag, Milan

Cesarani A, Alpini D, Barozzi S (1990) Electrical stimulation. In: Sacristan T, Alvarez-Vincent JJ, Bartual J, Antoli-Candela F (eds) The treatment of acute vertigo. Otorhinolaryngology, head and neck surgery. Proceedings of the XIV World Congress of Otorhinolaryngology, Madrid, 1989. Kugler-Ghedini, Amsterdam, Berkeley, Milan

Cesarani A, Alpini D, Barozzi S (1990) Neck electrical stimulation. The treatment of labyrinth acute vertigo. Riv It EEG Neurof Cl 13:1:55–61

Cesarani A, Alpini D, Boniver R, Claussen CF, Gagey PM, Magnusson M, Odkvist LM (eds) (1996) Whiplash injuries. Springer-Verlag, Milan

Claussen C-F (1969) Das Frequenzmaximum des kalorisch ausgelösten Nystagmus I als Kennlinienfunktion des geprüften Vestibularorgans. Acta Otolaryng (Stockh) 67:639

Claussen C-F (1969) Die quantitative Vestibularisprüfung – eine audiogrammanaloge Auswertung von Nystagmusbefunden (Schmetterlingsschema). Z Laryng Rhinol 48:938

Claussen C-F (1970) Der Kalorisationspendelinterferenztest (KPIT) 1. Mitteilung, Zeitschrift für Laryngologie, Rhinologie, Otologie 49

Claussen C-F (1970) Der Kalorisationspendelinterferenztest (KPIT) 2. Mitteilung, Zeitschrift für Laryngologie, Rhinologie, Otologie 49:326–332

Claussen C-F (1973) Butterfly vestibulometry, a practical evaluation scheme. Equilibrium Res 3:80–85

Claussen C-F (1974) El ciclograma de adaptacion. Otolaringologica, vol XI, pp 132–136

Claussen C-F (1979) The Rotatory Intensity Damping Test (RIDT) – a combined supraliminal and supramaximal nystagmus test. Acta Otorhinolaryng Belg 33:422–427

Claussen C-F (1980) Das belastungsabhängige Dysaequilibrium. Verh GNA 7

Claussen C-F (1981) Drei verschiedene Typen des vestibulären Recruitments. Verhlg GNA 8:487–504

Claussen C-F (1981) Schwindel – Symptomatik, Diagnostik, Therapie – ein Leitfaden für Klinik und Praxis. Edition m & p, Dr. Werner Rudat, Hamburg

Claussen C-F (1992) Der Schwindelkranke Patient – Grundlagen der Neurootologie und Äquilibriometrie. Edition m & p. Dr. Werner Rudat, Hamburg

Claussen C-F (1994) Vestibular compensation. Acta Otolaryngol (Stockh) Suppl 513:33–36

Claussen C-F (1995) Vestibular evoked potentials: a new frontier in equilibriometry. Acta Otolaryngol Suppl (Stockh) 520:113–116

Claussen C-F (ed) (1996) Giddiness and vestibulo-spinal investigations; combined audio-vestibular investigations. Experimental Neurootology. Excerpta Medica, Amsterdam

Claussen E, Claussen C-F (1976) Der Schwindelpatient aus der Sicht der HNO-Facharztpraxis. Verhdlg. der GNA, vol 5, pp 81–91

Claussen C-F, Claussen E (1986) Forschungsbericht Cranio-Corpo-Graphie (CCG) – ein einfacher, objektiver und quantitativer Gleichgewichtstest für die Praxis. Schriftenreihe des Hauptverbandes der gewerblichen Berufsgenossenschaften eV, St. Augustin

Claussen C-F, Claussen E (1988) Objective and quantitative vestibular spinal testing by means of computer-video-cranio-corpography. Adv Otolaryngol (Switzerland) 42:43–49

Claussen C-F, Claussen E (1991) Spatial stimulus interference upon ocular movements investigated by means of the Calorization Pendulum Interference Test (CPIT). Acta Otolaryngol Suppl (Stockh) 481:301–303

Claussen C-F, Claussen E (1995) Neurootological contributions to the diagnostic follow-up after whiplash injuries. Acta Otolaryngol Suppl (Stockh) 520:53–56

Claussen C-F, De Sa JV (1978) Clinical study of human equilibrium by electronystagmography and allied tests. Popular Prakashan, Bombay

Claussen C-F, Tato JM (1973) Equilibriometria practica. Edition Hasenclever & Cia, Buenos Aires

Claussen C-F, von Lühmann M (1976) Das Elektronystagmogramm und die neurootologische Kennliniendiagnostik. Edition m & p, Dr. Werner Rudat, Hamburg

Claussen C-F, von Schlachta I (1972) Butterfly chart for caloric nystagmus evaluation. Arch Otolaryng 96:371–375

Claussen C-F, Aust G, von Lühmann M (1973) Über das vestibuläre Recruitment und seine Darstellung mittels neuerer neurootologischer Kennlinienverfahren. HNO 21:196–198

Claussen C-F, Bergmann de Bertora JM, Bertora GO (1988) Otoneurooftalmologia. Springer-Verlag, Berlin Heidelberg New York, pp 1–124

Claussen C-F, von Schlachta I, Claussen E (1989) Tischtennis im Rahmen eines Übungsprogrammes für die Behandlung von Vertigo. Verhdgl. d. GNA, vol XI, pp 43–56

Claussen C-F, Claussen E, Patil NP, Schneider D (1989) The Rotatory Intensity Damping Test (RIDT). A combined clinical supraliminal and supramaximal rotational test. Acta Otolaryngol Suppl (Stockh) 468:313–316

Claussen C-F, Schneider D, Gfraas U, Hahn A (1991) Combined analysis of horizontal and vertical optokinetic nystagmus reactions by means of ENG and brain mapping. Acta Otolaryngol Suppl (Stockh) 481:221–223

Claussen C-F, Schneider D, Fraass U (1991) Therapeutical clinical models using the lower body negative pressure chamber for simulating vertebro-basilar insufficiency syndromes in humans. Acta Otolaryngol Suppl (Stockh) 481:548–550

Claussen C-F, Sajata E, Itoh A (eds) (1995) Vertigo, nausea, tinnitus and hearing loss in central and peripheral vestibular diseases. Excerpta Medica, Amsterdam

Claussen C-F, Constantinescu L, Kirtane MV, Schneider D (eds) (1996) Proceedings of the NES, vol XXIV, Elsevier Science BV, Amsterdam

Cohen H (1992) Vestibular rehabilitation reduces functional disability. Otolaryngology: Head Neck Surgery 107(N5):638–643

Cohen H (1994) Vestibular rehabilitation improves daily life function. Am J Occupational Ther 48(N10):919–925

Cohen H, Kanewineland M, Miller LV, Hatfield CL (1995) Occupation and visual vestibular interaction in vestibular rehabilitation. Otolaryngology: Head Neck Surgery 112(N4):526–532

Cohen H, Miller LV, Kanewineland M, Hatfield CL (1995) Vestibular rehabilitation with graded occupations. Am J Occupational Ther 49(N4):362–367

Craske B (1987) Perception of impossible limb position induced by tendon vibration. Science 71:738

Daleiden S (1990) Weight shifting as a treatment for balance deficits – a literature review. Physiother Can 48:81–87

Darlington CL, Smith PF (1996) Oscillopsia and dizziness resulting from gentamicin antibiotic treatment: a clinical note on the beneficial effects of vestibular rehabilitation therapy. N Z J Psychol V25(N2):24–28

Demer JL, Virre ES (1996) Visual-vestibular interaction during standing, walking and running. J Vest Res 6(4):295–313

DeSa-Souza S, Claussen C-F (1997) Modern concepts of neurootology. Prajakta, Bombay

Di Fabio RP, Andersen JH (1993) Effect of sway-referenced visual and somatosensory inputs on human head movement and postural patterns during stance. J Vest Res 3:409–417

Di Fabio RP (1995) Sensistivity and specificity of platform posturography for identifying patients with vestibular dysfunction. Phys Ther 75(4):290–304

Dilts R, Grinder J, Bandler R, Bandler LC, De Lozier J (1980) Neurolinguistic programming. Meta Publication, Cupertino, California

Dix DR (1974) Treatment of vertigo. Physiotherapy 60:380–386

Dix MR (1976) The physiological basis and practical value of head exercises in the treatment of vertigo. The Practitioner 217:919–924

Endsley MR, Rosiles SA (1995) Auditory localization for spatial orientation. J Vest Res 5:473–485

Epley J (1992) The canalith reposition procedure: for the treatment of benign paroxysmal vertigo. Otolaryngol Head Neck Surg 107:399–404

Epley J (1996) Particle repositioning for benign paroxysmal positional vertigo. Otolaryngol Clinic N Am 29:323–331

Fitzgerald G, Hallpike CS (1942) Studies in human vestibular function: 1. Observation on the directional preponderance of caloric nystagmus resulting from cerebral lesions. Brain 65:115–137

Foster CA (1994) Vestibular rehabilitation. Baillieres Clin Neurol 3(N3):577–592

Frederickson JM, Schwarz D, Kornhuber HH (1966) Convergence and interaction of vestibular and deep somatic afferents upon neurons in the vestibular nuclei of the cat. Acta Otolaryngol (Stockh) 61:168–188

Fukuda T (1961) Studies on human dynamic postures from the viewpoint of postural reflexes. Acta Oto-laryngol Suppl 161:1–52

Gagey PM (1988) La loi des canaux. Aggressologie 29:691–692

Ghez C (1991) Posture. In: Kandel ER, Schwartz JH, Jessel TM (eds) Principles of neural science. Elsevier, New York, pp 596–607

Gizzi M (1995) The efficacy of vestibular rehabilitation for patients with head trauma. J Head Trauma Rehabil 10(N6):60–77

Gluck MA, Rumelhart DE (eds) (1990) Neuroscience and connectionist theory. Lawrence Erlbaum Associates, Hillsdale, New Jersey

Goodwin GM, McClosely DI, Matthews PBC (1972) Proprioceptive illusions induced by muscle vibration: contribution by muscle spindle to prediction? Science 175:1382–1385

Goodwin GM, McClosely DI, Matthews PBC (1972) The contribution of muscles afferent to kinaesthesia shown by vibration induced illusions of movements and by the effects of paralysing joint afferents. Brain 95:705–707

Grateau P (1992) Critique de l'objectivite. Neuromedia, vol 11. Buk Club Neurosciences DEA, Marseille

Guedry FE, Rupert AH, Mcgrath BJ, Oman CM (1992) The dynamics of spatial orientation during complex and changing linear and angular acceleration. J Vest Res 2:259–283

Hadani I (1995) The spin theory – a navigational approach to space perception. J Vest Res 5:443–454

Hagbart KE (1973) The effect of muscle vibration in normal man and in patients with motor disorders. In: Desmedt JE (ed) New developments in electromyography and clinical neurophysiology. Karger, Basel, pp 428–443

Hahan A, Schneider D, Claussen CF (1995) Neurootological findings in patients with so-called Meniere-like disease. Acta Otolaryngol Suppl (Stockh) 20:134–135

Haken H (1983) Synergetics. An introduction. Springer-Verlag, Berlin, Heidelberg, New York

Hamann KF, Krausen C (1990) Clinical application of posturography – body tracking and biofeedback training. In: Brandt T, Paulus W, Bles W (eds) Disorders of posture and gait, Georg Thieme Verlag, New York, pp 295–298

Hamann R, Panzer V, Mekjavic I (1992) A comparison of postural therapeutic regimens using visual feedback of the center of gravity. In: Wollacott M, Horak F (eds) Posture and gait. Control mechanisms, Vol II. University of Oregon Books, Eugene, pp 376–379

Hamid MA (1994) Chronic dizziness – vestibular evaluation and rehabilitation. Cleveland Clinic J Med 61(N4):247–249

Henriksson NG, Jahneke JB, Claussen C-F (1969) Vestibular disease and electronystagmography. Press Company, Studentlitteratur, Lund, Sweden

Herdman SJ (1994) Vestibular rehabilitation. FA Davis, Philadelphia

Hikosaka O, Maeda M (1973) Cervical effects on abducens motoneurons and their interaction with vestibulo-ocular reflex. Exp Brain Res 18:512–530

Hinoki M, Ushio N (1975) Lumbomuscular proprioceptive reflexes in body equilibrium. Acta Otolaryngol Suppl 330:197–210

Hinoki M, Hine S, Okada S, Ishida Y, Koike S, Shizuku S (1975) Optic organ and cervical propioceptors in maintenance of body equilibrium. Acta Otolaryngol Suppl 330:169–184

Hirvonen TP, Aalto H, Pyykko I (1997) Stability limits for visual feedback posturography in vestibular rehabilitation. Acta Oto-Laryngologica (Suppl 529):104–107

Horak FB, Jonesrycewicz C, Black FO, Shumway-Cook A (1992) Effects of vestibular rehabilitation on dizziness and imbalance. Otolaryngology: Head Neck Surgery 106(N2):175–180

Horstmann GA, Dietz V (1990) A basic control mechanism: the stabilization of the center of gravity. Clin Neurophysiol 76:165–176

Howard IP (1997) Interactions within and between the spatial senses. J Vest Res 7:311–345

Igarashi M, Alford BR, Watanabe T, Maxiam PM (1969) Role of the neck proprioceptors for the maintenance of dynamic bodily equilibrium in the squirrel monkey. Laryngoscope 79:1713–1727

Karnath HO, Christ K, Hartjie W (1993) Decrease of controlateral neglect by neck muscle vibration and spatial orientation of the trunk midline. Brain 116:383–396

Kobayashi Y, Toshiaki, Kamio T (1988) The role of cervical inputs in compensation for unilateral labyrinthectomized patients. Adv Oto-Rhino-Laryng 42:185–189

Krebs DE, Gillbody KM, Riley PO, Parker SW (1993) Double-blind, placebo-controlled trial of rehabilitation for lateral vestibular hypofunction – preliminary report. Otolaryngology: Head Neck Surgery 109(N4):735–741

Jacobson P, Craig W, Newman C (1990) The development of the dizziness handicap inventory. Arch Otolaryngol: Head Neck Surg 116:425–427

Lackner JR (1988) Some proprioceptive influences on the perceptual representation of body shape and orientation. Brain 111:281–297

Lackner JR (1992) Multimodal and motor influences on orientation: implications for adapting to weightless and virtual environments. J Vest Res 2:307–322

Lackner JR (1992) Sense of body position in parabolic flight. Ann N Y Acad Sci 65:329–339

Lackner JR (1992) Spatial orientation in weightlessness environments. Perception 21:803–812

Lackner JR (1993) Spatial stability, voluntary action and causal attribution during self-locomotion. J Vest Res 3:15–23

Lackner JR (1993) Orientation and movement in unusual force environments. Psychol Sci:345–352

Lackner JR, Dizio P (1997) The role of reafference in recalibration of limb movement control and locomotion. J Vest Res 7:303–311

Lackner JR, Levine MS (1979) Changes in apparent body orientation and sensory localization induced by vibration of postural muscles: vibratory myoesthetic illusions. Aviation Space Environ Med 50:346–354

Latash ML (1993) Control of human movement. Human Kinetics Publishers, Champaign, USA

Ledoux A (1959) Les canaux semi-circulaires. Acta Otorhinolaryngol Belgica 12:2–3, 111–345

Lee DN, Lishman JR (1975) Visual proprioceptive control of stance. J Hum Mov Stud 1:87–89

Lempert T, Tiel-Wilck K (1996) A positional maneuver for treatment of horizontal-canal benign positional vertigo. Laryngoscope 106:476–478

Lindasy KW, Roberts TDM, Rosemberg JR (1976) Asymmetric tonic labyrinth reflexes and their interaction with neck reflexes in the decerebrate cat. J Physiol (London) 261:583–601

Luxon LM, Davies RA (eds) (1997) Handbook of vestibular rehabilitation. Singular Pub Group, San Diego

MacCloskey DI (1973) Differences between the senses of movement and position shown by the effects of loading and vibration of muscles in man. Brain Res (Amsterdam) 61:119–131

MacCloskey DI (1978) Kinesthesic sensibility. Physiol Rev 58:195–206

Maeda M (1979) Neck influences on the vestibulo-ocular reflex arc and the vestibulo-cerebellum. Prog Brain Res 50:551–559

Magnusson M (1994) Evaluation of brainstem-cerebellar posture control. In: Cesarani A, Alpini D (eds) Equilibrium disorders – brainstem and cerebellar pathology. Springer, Milan, pp 52–53

Manzoni D, Pompeiano O, Stampacchia G (1979) Tonic cervical influences on posture and reflex movements. Arch Ital Biol 117:81–110

Massion J, Woollacott MH (1996) Posture and equilibrium. In: Bronstein AM, Brandt T, Woollacott MH (eds) Clinical disorders of balance, posture and gait. Arnold Ed., London, pp 1–63

Mast F, Jarchow T (1996) Perceived body position and the visual horizontal. Brain Res Bull 40:393–398

Matin L, Wenxun L (1996) Multimodal basis for egocentric spatial localization and orientation. J Vest Res 5:499–518

McCabe BF, Ryu JH, Sekitami T (1972) Further experiments on vestibular compensation. Laryngoscope 82:381–396

Mendozzi L, Motta A, Barbieri E, Alpini D, Pugnetti L (1998) The application of the virtual reality to document coping deficits after a stroke. Cyberpsychol Behav 1:79–91

Mergner T, Anastasopoulos K, Becjer W, Deecke L (1981) Comparison of the modes of interaction of labyrinthine and neck afferents in the suprasylvian cortex and vestibular nuclei of the cat. In: Fuchs, Becker (eds) Progress in oculomotor research. Elsevier, Amsterdam, pp 343–350

Mergner T, Huber W, Becker W (1997) Vestibular-neck interaction and transformation of sensory coordiantes. J Vest Res 7:347–367

Mittelstaedt H (1997) Interaction of eye-head, and trunk-bound information in spatial perception and control. J Vest Res 7:283–303

Moore S, Wollacott MH (1993) The use of biofeedback devices to improve postural stability. Phys Ther Pract 2:1–19

Mruzek M, Barin K, Nichols DS, Burnett CN, Welling DB (1995) Effects of vestibular rehabilitation and social reinforcement on recovery following ablative vestibular surgery. Laryngoscope 105(N7):686–692

Nashner L (1994) Evaluation of postural stability, movement, and control. In: Hasson SM (ed) Clinical exercise physiology. Mosby, St. Louis, pp 67–85

Norré ME (1987) Rationale of rehabilitation treatment for vertigo. Am J Otolaryngol 8:31–35

Norrè ME (1990) Posture in otoneurology. Acta Otorhinolaryngol (Belgium) 44(N2–3):55–364

Paulus WM, Straube A, Brandt TH (1984) Visual stabilization of posture: physiological stimulus characteristics and clinical aspects. Brain 107:1143–1146

Poumarat G (1993) Les electrostimulateurs. Cah Kinesither 164:6:3–13

Previc FH (1992) The effects of dynamic visual stimulation on perception and motor control. J Vest Res 2:285–295

Pugnetti L, Alpini D, Cattaneo A, Barbieri E, Mendozzi L (1996) Computerized stabilometry in the assessment of some physiological after-effects of immersive virtual reality: a pilot study. In: Claussen CF, Constantinescu L, Kirtane MV, Schneider D (eds) Proceedings of the NES, vol XXIV, Elsevier Science BV, Amsterdam, pp 47–51

Raymond J, Sans A (1979) Projections somato-sensorielles dans les noyaux vestibulaires. Etude Electrophysiologique. J Physiol (Paris) 75:269–274

Redding GM, Wallace B (1993) Adaptive coordination and alignment of eye and hand. J Motor Behav 25:75–88

Regan D (1995) Spatial orientation in aviation: visual contributions. J Vest Res 5:455–471

Roll JP, Rol R (1988) From eye to foot: a proprioceptive chain involved in postural control. In: Amblard B, Berthoz A, Clarac F (eds) Posture and gait. Development, adaptation and modulation. Elsevier Science Publishers, Amsterdam, pp 155–166

Rosenbaum DA (1991) Human motor control. Academic Press, San Diego

Rudge P, Bronstein AM (1995) Investigations of disorders of balance. J Neurol Neurosurg Psych 59:568–578

Sachanska T, Haralanov H, Claussen C-F (1996) General and specific adaptation mechanisms under combined extreme effects. Significance for space biology and space medicine. Excerpta Medica, International Congress Series, vol 1133, Elsevier Publishers, Amsterdam, pp 361–367

Scherder EJ, Bouma A, Steen AM (1992) Influence of trancutaneous electrical nerve stimulation on memory in patients with dementia of the Alzheimer type J Clin Exp Neuropsychol (Netherlands) 14:951–960

Scherder EJ, Bouma A, Steen AM (1995) Effects of short-term trancutaneous nerve stimulation on memory and affective behaviour in patients with probable Alzheimer's disease. Behav Brain Res (Netherlands) 67:211–219

Schneider D, Hahan A, Claussen CF (1991) Cranio-corpography. A neurootological screening test. Acta Oto-Rhino-Laryngol (Belgium) 45:393–397

Schott E (1922) Über die Registrierung des Nystagmus und anderer Augenbewegungen vermittels des Seitengalvanometers. Dtsch Arch Klin Med 140:79–90

Semont A, Sterkers JM (1980) Reeducation vestibulaires. Les Cahiers D'Orl 15:305–376

Shepard NT, Telian SA (1995) Programmatic vestibular rehabilitation. Otolaryngology: Head Neck Surgery 112(N1):173–182

Shepard NT, Telian SA (1996) Practical management of the balance disorder. Patient Singular Pub Group, San Diego

Shepard NT, Smithwheelock M, Telian SA, Raj A (1993) Vestibular and balance rehabilitation therapy. Ann Otol Rhinol Laryngol 102(N3):198–205

Shumway-Cook A, McCollum G (1991) Assessment and treatment of balance deficits in the neurologic patients. In: Montgomery P, Connelly B (eds) Motor control. Theoretical framework and practical application to physical therapy. Chattanooga Corp., Chattanooga, TN, pp 123–138

Smithwheelock M, Shepard NT, Telian SA (1991) Physical therapy program for vestibular rehabilitation. Am J Otol 12(N3):218–225

Sterkers JM (1977) La methode du pointe de mire pour la reeducation anti-vertigineuse. Revue Laryng 535–538

Suarez H, Rosales B, Claussen CF (1992) Plastic properties of the vestibulo-ocular reflex in olivo-ponto-cerebellar atrophy. Acta Otolaryngol (Stockh) 112:589–594

Telian SA, Shepard NT (1996) Update on vestibular rehabilitation therapy. Otolaryngologic Clinics North Am 29(N2):359

Teramoto K, Sakata E, Yamashita H, Ohtsu K (1988) New Visual Suppression Test using post-rotatoric nystagmus II in the patients with cerebellar disease. In: Claussen C-F, Kirtane MV, Schlitter K (eds) Vertigo, nausea, tinnitus and hypoacusia in metabolic disorders. Excerpta Medica, Amsterdam, pp 485–488

Tokumasu K, Fujino A, Noguchi H (1993) Prolonged dysequilibrium in 3 cases with vestibular neuronitis – efficacy of vestibular rehabilitation. Acta Otolaryngologica (Suppl 503):39–46

Torok N (1948) Significance of the frequency in caloric nystagmus. Acta Otolaryng (Stockh) 36, 38

Ushio N, Hinoki M, Nakanishi K, Baron JB (1980) Role des propriocepteurs des muscles oculaires dans le maintain de l'équilibre du corps avec reference notamment au reflex cervical. Aggressologie 21:143–152

Watzlawick P, Beavin JH, Jackson DD (1967) Pragmatic of human communication. Norton & Co, New York

Wilson VJ, Maeda M, Franck JI (1975) Input from neck afferent to the cat flocculus. Brain Res 89:133–138

Yardley L, Luxon L (1994) Treating dizziness with vestibular rehabilitation. BMJ 308(N6939):1252–1253

Zennou-Azogui Y, Borel L, Lacour M, Ez-Zaher L (1993) Recovery of head postural control following unilateral vestibular neurectomy in the cat: neck muscle activity and neuronal correlates in Deiters' nuclei. Acta Oto-Laryngol (Stockh) (Suppl 509):19–23

Subject Index

Springer
and the
environment

At Springer we firmly believe that an international science publisher has a special obligation to the environment, and our corporate policies consistently reflect this conviction.
We also expect our business partners – paper mills, printers, packaging manufacturers, etc. – to commit themselves to using materials and production processes that do not harm the environment. The paper in this book is made from low- or no-chlorine pulp and is acid free, in conformance with international standards for paper permanency.

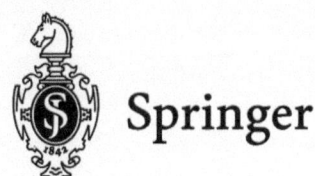 Springer

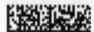